GRIEF
THE SILENT PANDEMIC

DOUG LAWRENCE

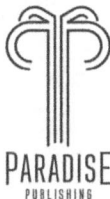

Paradise Publishing

Spring TX

2025

PARADISE
PUBLISHING

Publisher:
Paradise Publishing House
ParadisePublishingHouse.com
RogerLeslie.com

Grief: The Silent Pandemic / Doug Lawrence (1954 –)
    1. Bereavement—psychological aspects. 2. Bereavement—professional support. 3. Mentorship. 4. Mental health.

ISBN 978-1-941680-18-6 (perfect bound)
ISBN 978-1-941680-19-3 (eBook)

SUMMARY: After losing his beloved wife to cancer, a grief mentor shares personal and professional perspectives to make the difficult journey through grief easier for the bereaved and those who help them.

NOTE: No advice in this book is suggested as a replacement for direct, professional help. Consult your physician or mental health professional.

Dewey: 155.937

Book cover & interior design by – Deena Rae; E-BookBuilders, adaptation for ebook
About the Author photo by Andrea Norberg Photography

The paper used in this publication meets the requirements of the American National Standard for Permanence of Paper for Printed Library Materials Z39.48-1984.

For every book purchased, Paradise Publishing has a tree planted.

First edition.

Printed in the United States of America.

File version: 202411032.017

BOOKS BY DOUG LAWRENCE

The Gift of Mentoring
You Are Not Alone

c

CONTENTS

Books by Doug Lawrence c
Dedication .... g
Foreword 1
Introduction 3

Part I — Understanding Grief
Chapter 1 — What Is Grief? 11
Chapter 2 — The Facets Of Grief 21
Chapter 3 — The Impact Of Grief On Mental Health 29

Part II — Navigating The Grieving Process
Chapter 4 — Responses To Grief 41
Chapter 5 — Support For Grief 53
Chapter 6 — Grief Mentoring 59
Chapter 7 — Mentors As Bridges To Mental Health Support 79

Part III — Grief In Different Contexts
Chapter 8 — Grief And Youth 91
Chapter 9 — Grief In The Workplace 103
Chapter 10 — Grief And Trauma 115

Part IV — Moving Forward
Chapter 11 — Honoring Your Unique Grief Journey 125
Chapter 12 — Finding Meaning And Purpose 137
Chapter 13 — Supporting Others 143
Chapter 14 — Personal Progress 153

Conclusion 163
References 167
About The Author 169

DEDICATION

I am dedicating this book exclusively to my wife, Debra, who lost a battle with cancer in 2021. She was a dynamic individual who touched so many people. She was, and still is, my biggest cheerleader, standing by my side through thick and thin.

Debra would have offered her viewpoint(s) on this book if she was still here. She would have held me to task to tell the story the way she knew only I would.

Thank you, Debra, for your support, love, and guidance. I miss you dearly.

GRIEF
THE SILENT PANDEMIC

FOREWORD

H OW DO YOU FEEL WHEN someone "puts it all out there"?
What happens in your heart and stomach when you read
something so raw and genuine that you want to hug someone
you don't even know through the pages?

Why is it that, as humans, being our most human selves is so
unnatural and feels so filled with risk?

For those of you stepping into this book by Doug Lawrence
as the first opportunity to experience his gentle heart-wrenching
integrity, I say, "brace yourself." The voices of others that weave
through to build this story fill your mind and soul with a room full
of people that you get to know, care for, and love through the simple
act of them sharing their stories.

Grief is real. It is, of course, different for everyone, but given
that it lasts months, years, and decades, take a moment to consider
how often you have shared stories of grief with others. And as part of
that reflection, when someone shares their stories with you, how do
you resist that human urge to protect yourself from their pain—from
your pain—by physically or mentally slinking away?

Small wonder that mental health is taking its toll on society.

When I think about my beautiful millennial children, I wonder,
as a parent, if I have done enough to prepare them for the grief that
life holds. Did my divorce, my job loss, or uprooting them for yet
another move get the airtime that they needed to build the skills to
tackle life ahead? Or was I so focused on "being strong" and "being
positive" that I have deprived them of the opportunity to learn from
my sadness, from my weakness, from my grief? Death, job loss, loss
of a pet ... all potential triggers life will hand them. When I scan

1

the feeds in my social media, I see the world's violent indignation at job loss, the cold frozen messages of an unexpected death, and the trolling brick walls of opinion "This post doesn't belong here, don't be ridiculous" and I wonder, how do we build societal confidence in the need for learning and skill-building to support mental health, especially for life's most vulnerable moments?

It is time to break the silence. Time to lean into the discomfort. Time to embrace the learning and insight I've gained from every one of Doug's books, posts, and podcasts. I love the connection Doug has helped me see between the role of mentoring and mental health. As a society, we share stories of our trainers at the gym, the new workouts that we've tried, and the interesting new forms of exercise that ebb and flow in popularity. And we embrace the concept of maintaining and building on our physical health *before* a crisis—heart attack, high blood pressure, reduced mobility—forces us to make changes. Here is our opportunity, and the growing urgency, to do the exact same for our mental health and the mental health of those around us.

Grief is a crisis moment in a mental health journey. The stories Doug shares help us experience these very human responses in a safe and meaningful way. And they also signal for us the opportunity to tackle those future moments—unavoidable and sure to be unexpected moments—with some ideas for building understanding, coping skills, and the ability to support others in those moments of crisis.

Nature is not silent. The current popularity of forest bathing often touts itself as an avenue to sit in the silence of nature. What it actually does, in my view, is it blocks out the regular noise of day-to-day life to allow other sounds to be heard. It is time for us to consider the silence around us, to quiet our minds and environment enough to start healing the silent pandemic of mental health one moment, one interaction, one person at a time.

Yvonne Thevenot, MBA, ACMM, CCMP, CoA (IMC)
Independent Consultant, Change Management
Toronto, Canada

INTRODUCTION

WHEN I WROTE *You Are Not Alone*, I learned the importance of time alone to focus on writing. It was so easy to get pulled in multiple directions that I often cast aside the writing for another day. This time I wanted to change that. The nature of this book required me to zone in to get the job done. To facilitate this, I sought a writing space where I could finish the book. Unfortunately, carving out one at home wasn't enough. I needed a space where I could completely concentrate on my writing without any distractions.

I reserved an executive-style condo in a location that had meaning to me. To be honest, it had meaning to Debra and me. Our first posting as a married couple in the Royal Canadian Mounted Police was Invermere, just 15 kilometres down the highway from where I booked the condo in Radium Hot Springs, British Columbia. Debra had worked at the CIBC bank in Radium, so there are memories all around there for me. I took a large, framed picture of Debra and strapped it into the front seat where she would have sat and made my way to the condo. Every time I glanced over, I could see her sitting there with the biggest smile. Such fond memories of yesterday. I could not have made this journey or completed this book without her.

It seemed only fitting that this book would begin with a quick trip back in time. The relationship we shared was one of love and commitment to each other. This book is built upon the foundation of my experience with grief after losing Debra to cancer. Navigating this profound loss significantly affected my mental health. Working through my grief, I learned valuable lessons about my own life. More importantly, I learned about this *silent pandemic* that exists in our society.

Beyond my personal experiences, I am also a mentor who works with people struggling with grief. I know firsthand and vicariously that we need to appreciate relationships of love and commitment to each other. We need to understand how grief can impact our mental health and that grief is an integral part of our human journey.

While writing *You Are Not Alone,* I also realized that so much got left in the wings during the COVID-19 pandemic. We were so focused on dealing with the pandemic that we had put almost everything else on hold. Our mental health, mental well-being, and grieving the loss of a loved one or dear friend was far from many people's minds. People were consumed with the desire to stay alive during the pandemic. This also meant that supporting someone who was dying and their immediate family and/or friends was not front and center in their minds.

Unfortunately, the lack of attention to mental health and well-being was not created by the pandemic and/or its circumstances. It has been this way for a long time. People dealing with mental health challenges in silence have been doing so for decades, and we have continued to just push that aside. Sadly, the outcome of doing so has been tragic in many situations. Thus, our mental health situation has, in fact, reached a state of a pandemic whether we care to admit it or not. It is this pandemic that I refer to as the *silent pandemic.* Individuals are suffering, organisations are suffering, I am suffering. As a society, we have not been doing enough to alleviate this suffering.

Is Grief Part of the Mental Health Story?

The simple answer is yes. Grief is undeniably a part of the mental health story. Grief, a natural response to loss, can have a profound impact on an individual's mental well-being. It is a complex and multifaceted emotion that can manifest in various ways. It may encompass feelings of sadness, anger, guilt, and loneliness, among others. The grieving process is unique to each individual and can be influenced by factors such as the nature of the loss, personal coping mechanisms, and available support systems.

The correlation between grief and mental health is well-established. In society (our daily lives) we often either miss or simply overlook the link between the two. Studies have also shown that individuals who experience significant losses are at a higher risk of developing mental health problems. This is because grief can be an overwhelming and isolating experience, causing individuals to feel lost, hopeless, and disconnected from their support systems.

Because it is a normal and expected response to loss, grief is often overlooked as a mental health concern. Society often expects individuals to "move on" or "get over" their grief within a certain timeframe, failing to recognize that the grieving process is not linear and can last for an extended period.

However, when grief is not adequately addressed or processed, it can have severe consequences for an individual's mental health. Unresolved grief can lead to a state of prolonged mourning, characterized by persistent feelings of sadness, emptiness, and a lack of interest in daily activities. This can further develop into clinical depression, a serious mental health condition that requires professional intervention.

Grief can also trigger anxiety disorders, particularly when the loss is sudden or traumatic. Individuals may experience intense fear, worry, and panic attacks, as well as physical symptoms such as heart palpitations and difficulty breathing. In some cases, the trauma associated with loss can lead to developing PTSD, a mental health condition characterized by flashbacks, nightmares, and severe emotional distress.

The impact of grief on mental health can be further compounded by societal stigmas surrounding loss and mourning. Many individuals may feel pressure to hide their emotions or "be strong" in the face of loss, leading to a lack of proper support and resources. This can exacerbate feelings of isolation and contribute to the development of mental health problems.

Recognizing grief as a critical component of the mental health story is essential for promoting greater understanding, empathy, and support for those who are grieving. If we acknowledge the profound impact that loss has on an individual's well-being and provide access to appropriate resources and interventions as a society, we can help individuals navigate the complex terrain of grief and in turn mitigate the risk of long-term mental health consequences. Later on in this book, I will propose how this can be done.

WHY A SILENT PANDEMIC?

Mental health is a critical component of overall well-being, yet it is an aspect of health often overlooked and stigmatized in our society. The silent pandemic of mental health is a pervasive issue that affects individuals from all walks of life, and its impact is far-reaching and devastating.

The world is facing this silent pandemic primarily because so many lack awareness and understanding of mental health issues. Despite the fact that mental health problems are incredibly common, with one in five adults experiencing a mental illness in any given year, there is still a significant stigma attached to mental health. This stigma can prevent individuals from seeking the help they need, as they may feel ashamed, embarrassed, or afraid of being judged by others.

The COVID-19 pandemic exacerbated the silent pandemic of mental health. The isolation, uncertainty, and stress brought about by the pandemic took a significant toll on individuals' mental well-being. The disruption of daily routines, the loss of social connections, and the fear of contracting the virus all contributed to a rise in mental health issues such as anxiety, depression, and substance abuse. At its peak, the pandemic changed the way we grieved the loss of our loved ones, which further affected our mental health.

Debra passed away from cancer in 2021. Many people died from COVID and other illnesses and diseases as well, leaving loved ones to mourn their loss. However, mourning was not possible for many. The strategies put in place to keep us safe from the virus prevented us from mourning as we usually would. Lack of physical presence and support for many people during their grieving process impacted us significantly.

This brings me to a specific area where the silent pandemic of mental health is particularly evident—in the context of cancer and the grief that often accompanies it. Cancer is a devastating disease that affects not only the individual diagnosed but also their loved ones. The mental health impact of a cancer diagnosis can be profound, with individuals experiencing a range of emotions such as fear, anxiety, depression, and grief. The grieving process that follows the loss of a loved one to cancer can be especially challenging, as individuals may feel isolated and unsupported in their grief. The stigma surrounding both cancer and mental health can further compound this issue, making it difficult for individuals to seek the support they need. I found it especially difficult because of the COVID-19 restrictions in place when Debra died.

The consequences of the silent pandemic of mental health are far-reaching and devastating. When mental health issues go untreated, they can lead to a range of negative outcomes, including decreased quality of life, impaired relationships, and even suicide. In fact, suicide is the tenth leading cause of death in the United States. It is estimated that untreated mental illness costs the global economy over $1 trillion each year.

The silent pandemic also has significant implications for the workplace. Employees struggling with mental health issues may experience decreased productivity, increased absenteeism, and a higher risk of workplace accidents. This can have a significant impact on an organization's bottom line, as well as the overall morale and well-being of its workforce.

Clearly, addressing the silent pandemic of mental health requires a multi-faceted approach. This includes increasing awareness and education surrounding mental health issues, breaking down the stigma associated with seeking help, and continuously improving access to mental health services. It also requires a shift in societal attitudes towards mental health, recognizing that mental health is just as important as physical health and deserves the same level of attention and resources.

As a society, we must also recognize that mental health is not a one-size-fits-all issue. Each individual's mental health journey is unique, and we must create space for diverse expressions of mental health needs. This means fostering a culture of empathy, compassion, and understanding where individuals feel safe to share their experiences and seek the support they need.

In the chapters that follow, we will delve deeper into the complexities of grief and its impact on our lives. We will explore the various stages of grief, the unique challenges faced by different groups, and the importance of seeking support during the grieving process. Throughout the book, I will share personal anecdotes and insights from my own journey, as well as the experiences of others I have worked with who have experienced loss.

I have divided the book into four parts to provide a comprehensive understanding of grief and its many facets.

Part 1 lays the foundation by defining grief, examining the different types of grief, and exploring the profound impact it can have on our mental health.

Part 2 focuses on navigating the grieving process, offering strategies and tools for coping with the pain of loss, emphasizing the importance of seeking support, and highlighting the role of mentoring in providing guidance and companionship during this challenging time.

Part 3 explores grief in different contexts, such as the unique challenges faced by young people, the importance of organizational support for employees who are grieving, and the intersection of grief with other traumatic experiences.

Part 4 looks towards the future by drawing on the past. We will reflect on how grief can be transformative and lead to personal growth. We will also discuss the importance of using our own experiences to support others who are grieving, creating a ripple effect of compassion and understanding.

Throughout this book, my goal is to create a safe space for honest conversations about grief and mental health. In sharing my story and the stories of others whom I have had the privilege of mentoring, I hope to break down the stigma surrounding these topics and encourage readers to seek the support they need. I want to emphasize that grieving is a highly personal experience, and there is no "right" or "wrong" way to navigate this journey. What matters most is that we approach ourselves and others with compassion, patience, and understanding. Together, we can break the silence surrounding the mental health pandemic and create a world where no one has to suffer alone.

PART I

UNDERSTANDING GRIEF

CHAPTER 1

WHAT IS GRIEF?

I ENCOUNTERED THE PROFOUND DEPTHS OF grief when my beloved wife, Debra, passed away from cancer in 2021. Her battle was both swift and devastating; the cancer consumed her body with a vengeance. From the moment of her diagnosis in December 2020, I found myself grappling with the painful realization that my soulmate was slipping away.

I vividly recall that fateful moment in the emergency room when the doctor delivered the heart-wrenching news. The scans revealed lesions in Debra's lungs, liver, back, and brain. Though the doctor tried to maintain a positive outlook, deep down, I knew that my Debra was dying. As I sat there, holding her hand, I felt an emptiness grow within me, a void that soon deepened with each passing day.

The grief I experienced was multifaceted and all-consuming. It was a sadness so profound it felt like a constant physical weight upon my chest. It was a yearning for Debra's presence, for the life we had shared and the future we had dreamed of together. It was an anger at the injustice of it all, a desperate plea for her to be spared from this suffering.

While deeply personal, my experience is not unique. Grief is a shared human condition. Thus, it is both a natural and integral part of the human experience, a profound and often overwhelming response to loss. It is universal in its certainty and deeply personal in its unfolding.

At some point in our lives, each of us will inevitably face loss. When we lose someone or something we hold dear, we experience the complex mix of emotions, challenges, and eventual transformation that is grief. This loss can take many forms—the death of a loved one, the end of a cherished relationship, the loss of a job or a home, or even the loss of a long-held dream or sense of identity.

Grief is a multi-faceted response to loss that encompasses a range of emotions such as sadness, anger, helplessness, and more. It is not limited to emotional responses but can also affect an individual's physical health, mental health, social life, and overall well-being.

TYPES OF GRIEF

With the particulars of each person's grieving process may vary, certain commonalities can help us understand and navigate this difficult terrain. Grief experts have identified several types of grief, each with its own characteristics and challenges.

NORMAL GRIEF

Normal grief, sometimes referred to as uncomplicated grief, usually follows a progression of emotional stages that gradually lead to acceptance of the loss. People experiencing normal grief may go through a range of emotions including denial, anger, bargaining, depression, and finally acceptance. Though painful, normal grief is an adaptive response that allows the person to slowly reconcile with the reality of their loss and find a way to move forward.

COMPLICATED GRIEF

Complicated grief, or persistent complex bereavement disorder, is characterized by the extension of grief beyond what is considered a typical time frame. It involves prolonged periods of sadness, obsession with the deceased or the nature of the loss, and difficulties in resuming normal life activities. This form of grief can significantly impair one's ability to function in daily life and can lead to mental health problems such as depression or anxiety disorders.

ANTICIPATORY GRIEF

Anticipatory grief is the emotional response to an impending loss. When a loved one is terminally ill or ageing, one might begin to grieve long before the actual loss occurs. This type of grief includes mourning the impending loss, as well as grieving for the anticipated changes and adjustments that will need to be made in one's life. Anticipatory grief can also occur when facing a personal life-altering event such as the diagnosis of a terminal illness.

DISENFRANCHISED GRIEF

Disenfranchised grief refers to a loss that is not or cannot be openly acknowledged, socially validated, or publicly mourned. The griever is denied the social support ordinarily given to those who have experienced a loss. Common examples include the loss of a pet, the grief experienced by lovers when an extramarital affair ends, or the grief associated with the loss of a home or job. These losses can be just as significant to the individuals experiencing them but often lack the social recognition or support typically associated with grieving.

CUMULATIVE GRIEF

Cumulative grief occurs when an individual experiences multiple losses, either in quick succession or before fully processing a previous loss. This can lead to a compounding effect, where each new loss reactivates the pain of the others. Cumulative grief can be overwhelming, as the person may feel they are constantly in a state of mourning.

Collective Grief

Collective grief is experienced by a group or community. This occurs when members of a group, often bound by cultural ties, geographic location, or common goals, experience a shared loss. Examples include the grief experienced by a community after a natural disaster, terrorist attack, or the death of a public figure. Collective grief can also manifest on a larger scale as societal grief where large populations mourn a significant event such as a national tragedy.

When I reflect on my own journey grieving the loss of my wife, I see elements of many of these types: The anticipatory grief as Debra received her diagnosis and consequently battled cancer, the normal grief in the immediate aftermath of her passing, and even moments of complicated grief as I struggled to come to terms with a life without her by my side.

I also experienced disenfranchised grief at this loss because of the COVID-19 pandemic. The absence of the traditional mechanisms of solace and support, coupled with the enforced isolation, deepened the bottomless pit of grief I was in. The pandemic not only took away my wife, but also robbed me of the ability to mourn her in the traditional ways I had relied on in the past. When I lost my mother years earlier, I was able to find solace and support through the familiar rituals of grieving—the gathering of family and friends, the shared stories and memories, the communal acknowledgment of our loss. These rituals provided a sense of comfort and closure, helping me to navigate the complex emotions of grief.

Because Debra passed during the Covid-19 pandemic, I was denied these crucial avenues of support. The necessary restrictions on gatherings and travel meant I couldn't surround myself with the loving presence of family and friends. I couldn't hold the kind of funeral or memorial service I would have wanted to honor my wife's life and legacy. The pandemic stripped away these traditional ways of mourning, leaving me to grapple with my grief in isolation.

Absence of the usual rituals of grief made an already overwhelming process even more complex and challenging. Without the structure and support provided by these traditions, I felt completely untethered. In essence, the healing process became lonely and arduous, compounded by the universal stress and uncertainty of the pandemic.

Grieving in isolation, without the comforting presence of loved ones or the closure offered by shared rituals, was a profound challenge. It highlighted for me the importance of these traditions in helping us cope with loss, and how their absence can complicate and prolong the grieving process. Navigating grief during the Covid-19 pandemic reminded me of the vital role communal support and shared practices play in our healing, and how much more difficult the journey becomes when we are deprived of these sources of solace.

Using the definitions of grief that I presented earlier, I have been able to put some of what I experienced into words. That proved helpful for providing a framework for understanding grief. However, I've come to understand that they do not define the entirety of the grieving experience. Much of the grief I experienced cannot be articulated. Grief is messy, nonlinear, and deeply personal. It is a process of navigating a new normal, of learning to carry the weight of loss while still moving forward.

Throughout this journey, I will share more of my own story, the lessons I've learned, and the insights I've gained. While grief is an intensely personal experience, there is comfort in knowing we do not walk this path alone.

GRIEF INDICATORS

There are common signs, symptoms, and indicators that can help us identify and understand grief in ourselves and others. Recognizing these indicators is crucial for seeking and providing appropriate support during the grieving process. It's important to remember that grieving individuals have lost not only their loved one but also the shared future they had likely envisioned together. This loss of a shared future adds another layer to the complexity of grief in its various emotional, psychological, and physical manifestations.

The common signs and symptoms of grief we need to be cognizant of, whether as a person grieving or as someone helping someone else through grief, can be referred to as grief indicators. These include:

Shock and Disbelief

It's hard to accept death. We may feel numb and question whether the loss really happened. This isn't unusual. Some people have noted their initial reluctance even to notify others of a loss in case it turned out to be untrue. This can be a normal reaction to emotionally expect your person to call, write, or show up, even if, intellectually, you have accepted their death.

In my case, sitting in the ER with Debra and being given the diagnosis brought on feelings of shock and disbelief. I thought, *This was happening to others, but it couldn't be happening to us.*

Sadness

Profound sadness is a universal experience and can often lead to feeling alone or isolated. We sometimes believe that no one can understand the depth of our grief, which drives us deeper into sorrow. Sadness may lead to frequent crying, feelings of emptiness, and a sense of despair.

Guilt

We may feel guilt over things we said or did—or those we didn't and thought we should have. In cases of suicide, many people question whether they could have changed the outcome somehow. Yet nothing can stand in the way of death or a final decision made by someone else to die. Over time we have to acknowledge and accept that. Still, in the early days or months of grieving it's challenging to do.

ANGER

Regardless of how someone we loved died, anger often comes into play. We may be angry with the person for not being here anymore or with caregivers for not doing more. We may blame God, others, or ourselves. Sometimes we may not be able to direct our anger toward a specific source but find that daily, small injustices seem much more significant than they might have in the past. This is normal. It doesn't help for someone to tell us we must stop or let go of our anger. That will happen eventually as part of our process, on our timeline.

FEAR

A loss can trigger anxiety on many levels—fear of our mortality, losing those we love, and facing life without the person who died. It can include fear of the future and the uncertainty we may now feel about our life's plans, knowing that someone close to us has died.

PHYSICAL PAIN

We often think of grief as emotional, but it can also manifest physically. Symptoms can include nausea, fatigue, lowered immunity, weight loss or gain, insomnia, aches and pains, and more. Although it can be pretty difficult, it's essential to do what we can do to maintain our health during grief.

LONGING OR YEARNING

After a loss, it's common to experience a deep longing or yearning for the deceased. This can manifest as an intense desire to see, hear, or touch the person again. We may find ourselves reaching for the phone to call them, only to remember that they're no longer there. We might catch ourselves expecting them to walk through the door or to be in their usual spot at the dinner table. This longing can be particularly acute during special occasions or milestones that we normally would have shared with the deceased. It's a natural part of the grieving process, reflecting the depth of the attachment and the difficulty in adjusting to the loved one's absence.

DIFFICULTY CONCENTRATING

Grief can be all-consuming, occupying our thoughts and emotions to such an extent that it becomes difficult to concentrate on other things. We may find our minds constantly wandering to memories of the deceased or to thoughts about the loss. This can affect our ability to focus at work, to engage in conversations, or to complete everyday tasks. We may find ourselves forgetting things, misplacing items, or struggling to make decisions. This difficulty in concentration is a normal part of grieving, as our mind is trying to process and make sense of the loss. It's important to be patient with ourselves and to allow ourselves the time and space to grieve.

WITHDRAWAL AND ISOLATION

Some of us respond to loss by withdrawing from social contacts and isolating themselves. This may stem from a desire to avoid painful reminders of the loss, a fear of breaking down in front of others, or a feeling that no one else can truly understand what we're going through. We may decline invitations, avoid social gatherings, or spend more time alone. While some solitude can be helpful for processing grief, it's important to maintain connections with supportive others. Isolation can compound the pain of grief and lead to feelings of loneliness and depression. It's okay to take the time we need, but it's important to try staying connected to our support systems, even if it's just through brief check-ins or messages.

Grief is heterogeneous and can impact every aspect of our lives. If we are able to recognize the common signs and symptoms of grief, we can better understand our own experiences and the experiences of others who are grieving. This understanding is crucial for seeking and providing the necessary support, whether it be through mentors, professional help, or organizational resources. Acknowledging the complexity of grief and the various ways it can manifest, helps us create a more compassionate and supportive environment for ourselves and others who are navigating this challenging journey.

Besides recognizing indicators of grief, it can also be helpful to identify the stages of grief.

CHAPTER 2

THE FACETS OF GRIEF

THE JOURNEY THROUGH GRIEF IS complex and multifaceted. By exploring its various stages and manifestations, we can better understand what the grieving are facing throughout this often-arduous trek.

STAGES OF GRIEF

One of the most well-known frameworks for understanding grief is the concept of the "stages of grief," first introduced by psychiatrist Elisabeth Kübler-Ross in her groundbreaking 1969 book, *On Death and Dying*. Beyond recognizing these stages of grief, it can be helpful to understand what they entail and how they manifest in the lived experience of loss.

It's important to note that these stages are not a linear progression, but rather a framework for understanding the common emotions and challenges that arise during the grieving process. Not everyone will experience all of these stages, and the order and intensity of the stages can vary significantly from person to person.

Denial

Denial is often the first reaction to learning of a terminal illness or the death of a loved one. It is a normal defense mechanism that buffers the immediate shock of the loss, numbing us to our emotions. In this stage, the world becomes meaningless and overwhelming. Life makes no sense. In a state of shock, we may deny the difficult truth as a way to simply get through each day.

This was certainly true for me when Debra was diagnosed with cancer. Even though the doctor was clear about the severity of her condition, a part of me couldn't believe it was happening. I found myself going through the motions, but not really processing the reality of what we were facing.

Anger

As denial fades, the reality and the pain of the loss emerge. If we're not ready to accept it, we may focus on the unfairness of our loss. Anger is a necessary stage of the healing process. We may lash out at friends, family, or even complete strangers in an attempt to find someone or something to blame for our loss. We might also direct our anger at doctors for not saving our loved one, at our faith for allowing this to happen, or even at the deceased for leaving us. It's important to remember that beneath anger is pain. Anger is a secondary emotion; it's a response to feeling hurt, scared, or frustrated.

When Debra passed, I found myself feeling angry at the injustice of it all. I was angry at the cancer for taking her from me and at the world for continuing on when my own world had stopped.

Bargaining

At a point when we feel helpless and scared about loss, we often enter a bargaining stage. Bargaining is an attempt to regain control over a situation that feels uncontrollable. Often, we bargain with intangibles. In this stage, we may find ourselves making deals with a higher power or the universe, hoping that we can somehow reverse the loss. We bargain with our past and future. *If only I had …* or *What if I …* are common thoughts during this stage. We may bargain with the pain, hoping to postpone our grief and loss rather than face it head-on.

After losing Debra, I kept wondering if there was something more I could have done, some way I could have prevented her death if only I had been more insistent, more proactive. Common thoughts were: *If only we had sought medical attention sooner* or *If only I had been a better person.* At one point, I even bargained with God for my own life to be taken instead of hers.

DEPRESSION

As the reality of the loss begins to sink in, a deep sadness may ensue. When bargaining fails to provide relief, depression sets in. This is not a sign of mental illness; it is the appropriate response to a great loss. We withdraw from life, left in a fog of intense sadness, wondering, perhaps, if there is any point in going on alone. Morning may come, but we do not care. In the depths of despair, we see no hope, no future, no reason to continue. Holidays, anniversaries, and milestones can trigger a new cycle of grief and depression.

The weight of Debra's absence felt heaviest in these moments and still does.

ACCEPTANCE

This stage does not mean that the grieving individual is now "okay" or "over" the loss. Instead, acceptance is about acknowledging the loss and finding a way to move forward. In this stage, we accept the reality that our loved one is physically gone and that this new reality is the permanent one. We learn to live with it, not just to "get over it." We begin to live again, but we cannot do so until we have given grief its time.

For me, it is about learning to carry Debra's memory with me while also moving forward, about finding ways to honor our love and our life together while also embracing the life I have now. Since Debra's death, acceptance has been a gradual process. It still is. Some days, I fall back into the other stages and have to find my way back to the acceptance stage.

MANIFESTATIONS OF GRIEF

In addition to these five stages, it's important to acknowledge that grief can manifest it other ways as well. Those manifestations can be emotional, physical, or both.

EMOTIONAL MANIFESTATIONS

Grief can and does impact our general emotional health. Often it sparks changes in our moods and behaviors.

ANXIETY

Grieving frequently creates worry about what lies ahead. The loss might make us anxious about our own mortality, or we may worry excessively about the well-being of our other family members or friends. We may have a hard time concentrating. At its most intense, we might experience panic attacks or constant nervousness.

DEPRESSION

The profound sadness associated with grief can evolve into depression. A person may lose interest in things they once enjoyed and withdraw from social activities. They might struggle with feelings of worthlessness, experience a lack of appetite, and have difficulty finding pleasure in anything.

PHYSICAL MANIFESTATIONS

Grieving doesn't just affect the mind; it also has physical repercussions. The stress associated with loss can manifest in various ways.

Headaches

Tension and anxiety can cause frequent headaches. Headaches also tend to create similar symptoms as some emotional responses to grief, such as lack of focus and isolation. Such compounded effects of grief can make the struggle through it even more difficult.

Nausea

Grieving individuals might feel physically ill. Commonly, sadness or anxiety from grieving can play havoc on the digestive and gastrointestinal systems. The most common effects of grief may be stomach aches or loss of appetite.

Weakened Immune System

Chronic stress due to grief may weaken the immune system, making us more susceptible to illness. A combination of emotional and physical illness can spiral into an even greater struggle to overcome either.

Fatigue

A constant sense of tiredness and lack of energy may persist. Fatigue may be exacerbated by depression and could even lead to sleep disturbances.

Sleep Disturbances

Grief is frequently associated with different forms of sleep disruptions. From individual nightmares to chronic insomnia, sleep disturbances can lead to mental and physical exhaustion.

Psychological Manifestations

Sometimes the impact of grief, and how we handle or try to avoid handling it, can impact both our emotional and physical states simultaneously. At its direst, it might lead to life-altering behaviors or illnesses.

SUBSTANCE ABUSE

The grieving sometimes turn to alcohol and/or other substances to avoid facing the pain of grief or even to dull its impact. Unfortunately, when the immediate sense-dulling effects wear off, we often face even deeper sadness or loss, or physical symptoms that keep us from moving toward wellness. Left unchecked, indulgence can lead to abuse of alcohol or drugs, or dependency on substances. If abuse or dependency spill into addiction, we are left with seemingly insurmountable challenges to find balance and peace in our lives.

POST-TRAUMATIC STRESS DISORDER (PTSD)

Grief, especially in cases of sudden or violent loss, can lead to PTSD. Beyond more common features of grief described in the types and stages of grief, PTSD encompasses some unique characteristics.

When we suffer from PTSD, we are more quickly and profoundly impacted by certain sights, sounds, or smells. These triggers spark intense emotional and physical reactions. We might also suffer from flashbacks where we relive the traumatic event repeatedly in our minds. PTSD can ignite hyperarousal, a state where we may feel constantly on edge, are easily startled, and have difficulty sleeping. Finally, PTSD can force us into an even more pronounced state of avoidance, where we attempt to stay clear of places, people, or things that remind us of the traumatic event.

We will have our own journey through grief. Some of us may experience many of the stages and manifestations of grief exactly as described above. Some may recognize only some stages and know the struggles of some manifestations. As we navigate the stages of grief, it's crucial to remember that there is no "right" or "wrong" way to grieve. Some of us will wear our emotions on our sleeve; others will keep our feelings close to our heart. Some will find solace in talking about our loss; others will prefer to grieve privately. While some of us will need to slow down and allow ourselves to simply feel, some will find comfort in keeping busy. What's most important is that we grant ourselves grace and patience as we navigate this difficult journey.

CHAPTER 3

THE IMPACT OF GRIEF ON MENTAL HEALTH

O NE OF THE MOST DEVASTATING contributors to the mental health pandemic is unresolved grief. Yes, grief is a natural response to loss, but when it is not properly addressed, it can severely impact mental health.

We have already established that grief is a deeply personal experience that can manifest in different ways for different people. It can encompass a wide range of emotions, including sadness, anger, guilt, and loneliness. It can also lead to physical symptoms, such as fatigue, insomnia, and changes in appetite.

When we lose someone or something significant, it's normal to go through some or all the stages of grief. However, grief becomes particularly problematic when it is complicated or unresolved .

Complicated grief is a persistent and debilitating form of grief that does not improve with time. It's characterized by intense longing, intrusive thoughts, avoidance of reminders, and a sense of meaninglessness.

Unresolved grief can lead to depression, anxiety, substance abuse, and even suicidal ideation. It can affect every aspect of life, from our relationships and work to our physical health and overall quality of life.

Only by addressing the importance of mental health can we prevent natural and gradually abating grief from becoming complicated or unresolved.

DEFINING MENTAL HEALTH

Mental health in an umbrella term that covers various aspects of our cognitive, emotional, and social well-being. Essentially, it's the amalgamation of our thoughts, emotions, and social interactions, and how these elements interplay in our lives. It influences how we think, feel, and behave, and determines how we handle stress, relate to others, and make choices.

Mental health is more than just the absence of mental disorders. It includes having a positive sense of self, healthy relationships, and the ability to cope with life's challenges. Mental health is important at every stage of life, from childhood and adolescence through adulthood and aging. Three different aspects of mental health contribute to our overall wellbeing at all stages of life.

COGNITIVE ASPECT

Cognition refers to our mental processes, including memory, perception, problem-solving, and decision-making. It's about how we process information, how we learn, and how we utilize the knowledge acquired.

EMOTIONAL ASPECT

The emotional aspect of mental health encompasses our feelings and how we manage them. Emotional well-being involves effectively handling emotions such as happiness, sadness, anger, fear, and frustration. While more commonly associated with our ability to cope with negative emotions, it also includes the ways we express positive emotions.

SOCIAL ASPECT

The social dimension of mental health concerns our interactions with others and the surrounding environment. It includes our ability to establish and maintain satisfying relationships, work in groups, and contribute to the community.

WHY MENTAL HEALTH MATTERS

Despite its importance, mental health often receives only cursory attention in our societal discourse. When mental health is addressed, its issues are frequently stigmatized, misunderstood, or simply not given the attention they deserve. This neglect has led to the "silent pandemic" of mental health.

The term "silent pandemic" is particularly apt when discussing mental health because, unlike physical illnesses, mental health struggles are often invisible. We can suffer profoundly on the inside while presenting a façade of normalcy to the world. This invisibility, coupled with the stigma surrounding mental health, leads to a vast number of people suffering in silence.

In order to create a society that prioritizes good mental health, we must address this stigmatization, misunderstanding, and lack of attention to our mental health issues. Because good mental health serves as a foundation for a fulfilling and productive life, we must make it a cornerstone of our societal awareness.

It plays a significant role in our ability to function effectively and live a life that includes happiness and a sense of meaning. Good mental health enables us to have both everyday and exceptional human experiences. Only with it can we:

ENJOY LIFE

When in good mental health, we can savor various experiences, activities, and relationships, which contribute to a higher quality of life. This enjoyment is integral to sustaining a sense of contentment and happiness.

LIVE A BALANCED LIFE

Achieving psychological resilience requires finding a balance among work, leisure, relationships, and personal time. This balance enables us to handle stressors effectively and participate in life without feeling overwhelmed or stretched too thin.

ADAPT TO ADVERSITY

Life can be unpredictable and challenging. Mental health resilience is crucial in adapting to setbacks, traumas, and stress. A strong mental state helps us overcome obstacles and transform challenges into opportunities.

FOSTER RELATIONSHIPS

Mental health affects how we interact with others. Being mentally healthy can lead to building deeper, more meaningful relationships with family, friends, and colleagues.

MAKE MEANINGFUL DECISIONS

When our mental health is optimal, we have a clearer, more focused mindset. This clarity allows us to make decisions based on rational thinking rather than being overly influenced by uncontrollable emotions. This focused, rational state empowers us to be:

PRODUCTIVE

Good mental health can significantly boost productivity and performance in various aspects of life, including work and education. When mentally healthy, we are more likely to be motivated, focused, and efficient in our tasks.

SELF-AWARE

Prioritizing mental health often involves introspection and self-reflection. This process can lead to increased self-awareness, enabling individuals to better understand their emotions, thoughts, and behaviors. Self-awareness is crucial for personal growth and self-improvement.

CREATIVE

A healthy mental state can foster creativity and innovation. When not burdened by excessive stress or mental health issues, we are more likely to think creatively, generate new ideas, and approach problems from different perspectives.

RESILIENT

Focusing on mental health can help us develop resilience— the ability to bounce back from adversity. Resilient people are better equipped to cope with stress, adapt to change, and overcome challenges.

GRIEF'S INFLUENCE ON DAILY LIFE

Mental health is not an isolated aspect of our lives. Because it is interwoven with every action, decision, and interaction, it influences daily life in various ways.

STRESS MANAGEMENT

Our mental state significantly influences how we deal with stress. Good mental health provides the tools necessary to tackle stressors head-on, rather than allowing them to overwhelm us.

COMMUNITY ENGAGEMENT

When individuals prioritize their mental health, it not only benefits them personally, but also contributes to the overall well-being of society. Mentally healthy individuals are more likely to engage in prosocial behaviors, such as volunteering, and to be active and positive contributors to their communities.

Personal Impact

Our mental health shapes how we perceive the world around us. It affects our attitudes, beliefs, and interpretations of events, which in turn influences how we respond to different situations in our daily lives.

Physical Health

Mental and physical health are closely linked. A healthy mental state can lead to better physical health outcomes and vice versa.

Work Performance

Our mental state can greatly affect our performance at work. Good mental health contributes to increased productivity, better concentration, improved problem-solving abilities, and more harmonious professional relationships.

Self-Esteem

Our mental health is closely tied to our self-esteem and self-worth. A healthy mental state promotes a positive self-image, self-acceptance, and self-confidence. Those intrapersonal qualities empower us to pursue our goals and color our interpersonal interactions with individuals, groups, and the world at large.

Emotional Regulation

Mental health sets the gauge for our ability to regulate and manage our emotions. It influences how we respond to and express our feelings. Even further, it determines how we cope with and bounce back from negative emotional experiences.

Growth

A healthy mental state fosters a growth mindset and openness to new experiences. It encourages learning, adaptability, and personal development, allowing us to continually evolve and improve.

QUALITY OF LIFE

Ultimately, mental health has a profound impact on our overall quality of life. It influences our sense of fulfillment, life satisfaction, and general well-being. Good mental health allows us to engage with life fully, find meaning and purpose, and thrive in the face of challenges.

FAMILY DYNAMICS

Mental health plays a crucial role in family dynamics, especially parenting. It sets the stage for how we interact with our children, our partners, and other family members, as well as how we handle the challenges and joys of family life. Good mental health promotes positive parenting practices and healthy family relationships.

ACADEMIC PERFORMANCE

For students, mental health is a primary determiner of academic performance. It affects concentration, memory, motivation, and the ability to manage stress and anxiety related to studies. Prioritizing mental health can lead to improved learning outcomes and academic success.

RISKS AND DECISIONS

Mental health ties in directly with our ability to assess risks and make sound decisions. It directs our judgment, our impulse control, and our ability to consider long-term consequences. Good mental health promotes responsible and balanced decision-making.

Addiction Prevention

Mental health and substance use disorders often go hand-in-hand. Poor mental health can increase the risk of developing substance use problems. In turn, substance use can exacerbate mental health issues. Maintaining good mental health is crucial for preventing and recovering from addictive behaviors.

Life Transitions

Mental health plays a significant role in navigating life transitions, such as starting a new job, getting married, dealing with loss, becoming a parent, or retiring. Good mental health enables us to adapt to change, cope with new challenges, and find meaning and purpose in new stages of life.

Spiritual Well-Being

For many individuals, mental health is connected to spiritual well-being. A healthy mental state can facilitate a deeper connection with one's spiritual beliefs, values, and practices. That connection can lead to a greater sense of purpose, meaning, and inner peace.

Financial Advantages

Investing in mental health can lead to reduced healthcare costs in the long run. When mental health issues are addressed early and effectively, it can prevent the development of more severe and costly conditions.

Maintaining good mental health is a continuous journey that requires self-awareness, commitment, and a holistic approach, especially when navigating the profound impact of grief. Ultimately, addressing the silent pandemic of mental health requires a shift in our collective understanding. We must make mental well-being a top priority, particularly in the context of grief. By giving mental health the same attention and resources that we give physical health, we can create a culture that validates and supports the unique challenges of the grieving process.

Our task is two-fold. We should first recognize the profound impact grief has on our mental health. With that awareness we can then embrace strategies to cope with and heal from loss. Those strategies, both generally effective and personally adaptive, will enable us to work towards building a society that is more emotionally resilient, empathetic, and equipped to support one another through life's most difficult moments. Mental health is a precious asset that deserves our attention and care, especially during times of grief.

PART II

NAVIGATING THE GRIEVING PROCESS

CHAPTER 4

RESPONSES TO GRIEF

DEBRA TOUCHED SO MANY LIVES because she was such an outgoing "people person" and had a heart that was so big. I wondered all the time how someone could love as deeply as she did. Her influence was far-reaching, but her most powerful impact was on me. She helped me discover who I really am. I know that the love we shared is so deep it is a gift unto itself. She was and always will be an amazing woman, and I am truly blessed to have spent the time with her that I did. My sadness continues because I did not get the full benefit of Debra as she was stolen from me far too early. It truly was not fair.

How do I deal with the loss of all this love? At times I need a good cry, and I have learned that I need not be ashamed of my emotions. It's okay to weep, and it's okay to be sad. Trying to be strong for your family isn't being truthful to yourself and to others. They need to know you are in a state of grief; you were the one who lost your most beloved treasure, your partner that was to be for life.

All your plans have been stolen and you are left to rethink the rest of your life without that person. The inability to follow through pokes at your managing of grief as memories remind you of how it was and how it will never be. Traditions can be modified but never replaced. For me, a tradition without Debra is not a tradition. Now I am dealing with so much more and still don't understand "why." I miss the intimacy that was a part of who Debra really was. I remember the first time I met her mom. On a walk, she told me Debra was a person who needed lots of love and that in return she would give as much as she got. That was never far from the truth. I gave all that I could, and I got back tenfold from Debra. That made her passing especially hard to deal with as there was now this gaping hole I had to struggle to fill.

COPING WITH GRIEF

There is hope, however, for we can use strategies to cope with grief. Of course, this will be unique to each individual. However, here are some strategies that I suggest might be helpful:

ALLOW YOURSELF TO FEEL YOUR EMOTIONS

One of the most important aspects of coping with grief is giving yourself permission to feel the full range of emotions that come with loss. These may include:

SADNESS

Acknowledging and expressing the deep sorrow that accompanies loss is a crucial part of the grieving process. Allow yourself to cry, and don't feel ashamed of your tears.

ANGER

It's common to feel anger towards the situation, the loved one who died, or even towards yourself. Recognize this as a normal part of grief and find healthy ways to express it, such as through physical activity or talking with a trusted friend.

GUILT

Thoughts of "what if" and "if only" often plague those who are grieving. Understand that these feelings are common. Try not to dwell on things that cannot be changed.

LONELINESS

The absence of your loved one can create a profound sense of loneliness. Reach out to others for support and companionship, even when it feels difficult.

JOURNAL

Writing about your thoughts, feelings, and memories can be a powerful tool for processing your grief. Journaling can:

PROVIDE A SAFE SPACE TO EXPRESS YOUR EMOTIONS

A journal is a private, non-judgmental outlet for your grief.

HELP YOU MAKE SENSE OF YOUR EXPERIENCES

Writing can help you organize your thoughts and gain new insights into your grief journey.

HONOR YOUR LOVED ONE

Use your journal to record special memories, stories, or lessons learned from your loved one. Set aside dedicated time each day to write, and don't worry about grammar or structure. The act of putting your thoughts on paper is what matters.

PRIORITIZE SELF-CARE

Grief can take a significant toll on both physical and mental health. Prioritizing self-care is essential for managing the stress and emotional turmoil of loss. Several self-care activities can net impressive, comforting results.

Exercise Regularly

Physical activity can help boost mood, reduce stress, and improve sleep. Aim for at least 30 minutes of moderate exercise most days of the week.

Eat a Healthy Diet

Nourish your body with a balanced diet rich in fruits, vegetables, whole grains, and lean proteins. Avoid excessive alcohol or substance use, which can exacerbate grief symptoms.

Get Enough Sleep

Grief can disrupt sleep patterns. Adequate rest is crucial for emotional and physical resilience. Aim for 7-9 hours per night and practice good sleep hygiene.

Practice Relaxation Techniques

Deep breathing, meditation, or gentle yoga can help calm the mind and reduce stress.

Remember, self-care is not selfish. Taking care of yourself puts you in a better position to navigate your grief and support others who may also be grieving.

Seek Support

Grief can feel isolating, but it's essential to remember that you don't have to face it alone. Seeking support from others can provide comfort, validation, and a sense of connection during this difficult time. Some sources of support include:

FRIENDS AND FAMILY

Reach out to loved ones who can offer a listening ear, practical help, or a shoulder to cry on.

A MENTOR

A mentor can be a trusted friend, family member, or someone from a professional mentoring program. Mentors, especially those who have experienced grief themselves, can provide valuable support and guidance. They can share their own coping strategies, offer a non-judgmental listening ear, and help you navigate the complex emotions and challenges that come with grief.

SUPPORT GROUPS

Joining a grief support group can provide a sense of community and understanding among others who have experienced similar losses.

PROFESSIONAL COUNSELING

A therapist or counselor specializing in grief can offer additional guidance and coping strategies tailored to your unique needs.

A FAITH OR SPIRITUAL COMMUNITY

For those who find comfort in religion or spirituality, reaching out to a faith leader or spiritual community can provide solace and support during times of grief. Many religious and spiritual organizations offer grief support services, such as counseling, prayer groups, or healing rituals, which can help individuals find meaning and comfort in their beliefs.

Don't hesitate to ask for help when you need it. Allowing others to support you is a sign of strength, not weakness.

HONOR YOUR LOVED ONE'S MEMORY

Finding ways to celebrate and honor your loved one's life can bring comfort and can help maintain a sense of connection. You might:

CREATE A MEMORY BOOK OR BOX

Collect photos, letters, or other mementos that hold special meaning and compile them into a tribute to your loved one.

PARTICIPATE IN MEANINGFUL RITUALS

Engage in activities or traditions that were important to your loved one. Volunteering for a cause they believed in or cooking their favorite meal can be richly comforting.

SHARE STORIES

Keep your loved one's memory alive by sharing stories and memories with others who knew and cared for them.

Like grieving them, honoring your loved one's memory is a deeply personal process. Choose activities that feel authentic and meaningful to you.

PRACTICE MINDFULNESS AND SELF-COMPASSION

Mindfulness and self-compassion are powerful tools for navigating the challenges of grief. Mindfulness involves being present in the moment and observing your thoughts and feelings without judgment. Self-compassion entails treating yourself with kindness while recognizing that grief is a difficult and painful experience. Here are some ways to practice mindfulness and self-compassion:

FOCUS ON THE PRESENT

When grief feels overwhelming, bring your attention back to the present moment. Notice your breath, your surroundings, and the sensations in your body.

ACKNOWLEDGE YOUR PAIN

Accept that your pain is valid. Many times throughout the grieving process, it's okay not to be okay.

TREAT YOURSELF WITH KINDNESS

Speak to yourself as you would to a dear friend who is suffering. Use that same compassion in your silent thoughts. Let your words and thoughts offer comfort and understanding.

ENGAGE IN SELF-CARE

Regularly engage in activities that bring you a sense of peace and comfort. These diversions or consistent practices can be very simple, such as taking a warm bath, reading a favorite genre of book, or spending time in nature.

Remember, grief is a process, not a destination. Be patient with yourself and trust that healing will come with time.

FIND MEANING AND PURPOSE

In the midst of grief, it can be helpful to find ways to create meaning and purpose. You can:

REFLECT ON YOUR LOVED ONE'S LEGACY

Consider the values, lessons, or qualities that your loved one embodied. Further, think about how you can carry those forward in your own life.

Help Others

Engaging in activities that help others can provide a sense of purpose and connection. Effective practices can include volunteering or even supporting others who are grieving.

Set New Goals

Life usually feels different after a loss. Setting new goals for yourself can help you find direction and motivation.

Finding meaning and purpose is a highly individual process and not everyone will. What brings a sense of significance to one person may not resonate with another.

While the strategies and tools outlined in this chapter can be immensely helpful, it's essential to recognize that grief does not have a clear endpoint. Healing happens gradually, and setbacks are a normal part of the journey. Be patient with yourself, seek support when needed, and trust that you will find your way forward.

The Case Study

Before moving on to the next chapter, I would like us to explore a case study as it relates to coping with grief. More specifically, the case study is intended to delve into the grief management techniques employed by a person named Sarah, who endured intense grief following the unexpected death of her spouse. By scrutinizing Sarah's path and the strategies she utilized to steer through her sorrow, we can glean valuable knowledge about practical coping tactics that might serve others grappling with analogous circumstances.

Here's background for the case: Sarah, a woman in her late thirties, faced the heartbreaking loss of her husband due to an unforeseen accident. Their shared life spanned over 12 years of marriage, and they were blessed with two children. The sudden demise of her spouse plunged Sarah into profound despair, engulfed by a torrent of emotions and a struggle to find purpose in her existence. Consumed by grief, she turned to a grief counsellor for assistance and adopted several coping techniques to guide her through her grieving journey. Her efforts can help others who grieve navigate their own difficult journey.

UTILIZE COPING STRATEGIES

While different strategies work for different people, using Sarah's journey as an example may help to appreciate the challenges and benefits of taking steps that may fit our needs as we grieve. Often we don't know what will help us most until we try it.

SEEK PROFESSIONAL ASSISTANCE

Acknowledging her need for expert intervention, Sarah initiated her healing journey by participating in therapeutic sessions with a grief counsellor. These sessions provided her with a safe and non-judgmental platform to vent her emotions and fears. The guidance offered in these sessions helped her better understand and manage her grief while also equipping her with personalized coping strategies to suit her unique circumstances.

CULTIVATE A SUPPORTIVE NETWORK

Sarah actively contacted her friends, family members, and grief support groups. She established connections with individuals who had suffered similar losses, finding comfort in sharing her personal feelings and experiences with them. This network served as a source of empathy and comprehension, effectively alleviating her sense of loneliness and promoting a feeling of communal solidarity.

TRY EXPRESSIVE WRITING

Sarah discovered an emotional refuge in expressing her innermost thoughts and sentiments through writing in a personal journal. This expressive writing served as a cathartic tool that allowed her to navigate her grief, delve into her emotions, and gain a more profound understanding of her thoughts. It became a therapeutic outlet for her, facilitating emotional release and imparting clarity to her feelings.

Prioritize Self-Care

Once she realized the critical role of self-care in her grieving process. Sarah made it a priority. She incorporated activities that induced comfort and enhanced her physical and mental well-being. Regular physical exercise, balanced nutrition, meditation practices, and sufficient sleep became an integral part of her routine. Those various activities all contributing to rejuvenating her physical strength and emotional resilience.

Engage in Therapeutic Activities

Sarah became involved in activities that encouraged healing and served as a healthy distraction from her persistent grief. She regularly took part in a bereavement support group. Occasionally she attended workshops focused on grief management. She increasingly explored creative expressions such as art therapy and music therapy. These activities fostered a renewed sense of purpose, stimulated social interaction, and promoted personal development.

Pursue Meaning and Purpose

As part of her coping strategy, Sarah undertook a quest to discover a renewed sense of meaning and purpose in her life post-loss. While delving into spirituality, she embarked on introspective journeys and contemplated existential questions prompted by her loss. This explorative process helped her unearth new sources of inspiration. Along the way she developed a deeper understanding of life and fostered a more profound appreciation of her existence.

ASSESS THE RESULTS AND IMPACT

As Sarah utilized these coping mechanisms, she noticed a gradual progression towards healing and personal development within her grieving journey. Despite the enduring ache of loss, she cultivated resilience. Through her new, deeper self-awareness, she revived a sense of purpose in her life. These coping methods empowered her to grapple with the intricate emotional facets of grief and adjust to her transformed circumstances.

THE CASE STUDY OUTCOMES

Conclusion: This case study underscores the critical role of employing practical coping techniques during the grieving process. Sarah's journey exemplifies how actions such as securing professional assistance, cultivating a supportive network, prioritizing self-care, partaking in therapeutic activities, articulating emotions through writing, and pursuing a sense of meaning and purpose can substantially aid in the healing process. By identifying and embracing these strategies, those traversing the path of grief like Sarah can discover effective methods to manage their feelings to promote healing. The result is ultimately reconstructing a life amidst loss.

CHAPTER 5

SUPPORT FOR GRIEF

IN THE PREVIOUS CHAPTER, I briefly mentioned seeking support as a way of dealing with grief. In this chapter, we will explore the various ways in which reaching out and finding help can support mental health and well-being during the grieving process. Then in the chapter that follows, we will place particular focus on the role of mentoring in providing guidance and support.

SEEK SUPPORT

One of the most significant challenges of grieving is the sense of isolation and loneliness that often accompanies the loss of a loved one. As we grieve, it is not uncommon to feel disconnected from others, even when surrounded by family and friends. This is where seeking support becomes vital. Reaching out to others holds the potential for many benefits.

FIND A SAFE SPACE TO EXPRESS EMOTIONS

Finding a safe and supportive environment to express the complex and often overwhelming emotions that come with loss is challenging. We might feel pressured to "stay strong" or "move on" before we are ready, leading to the suppression of emotions and a sense of isolation. Seeking support, whether through professional help, support groups, or mentoring relationships, can provide a safe and non-judgmental space to express emotions openly and honestly.

Gain Validation and Understanding

Grief can be a profoundly lonely experience, particularly when those around us have not experienced a similar loss. Seeking support from others who have gone through the grieving process can provide a sense of validation and understanding. Knowing that others have experienced similar emotions and challenges can help us feel less alone and more supported in our journey.

Learn Coping Strategies

Grieving is a complex and often unpredictable process, and it can be difficult to know how to cope with the various emotions and challenges that arise. Seeking support from professionals, such as therapists or grief counselors, can provide valuable tools and strategies for managing our grief. Support groups and mentoring relationships can also offer practical advice and guidance based on the experiences of others who have gone through similar losses.

Address Related Challenges

Grief can often be compounded by related challenges, such as financial strain, legal issues, or family conflicts. Seeking support from professionals or organizations specializing in these areas can help us overcome these hurdles more stridently, reducing stress and allowing us to focus on our emotional healing.

FIND THE RIGHT SUPPORT

While seeking support is crucial for navigating the grieving process, it is important to recognize that not all forms of support will be equally beneficial for everyone. The key is to find the support that feels most comfortable and effective for your unique needs and circumstances.

PROFESSIONAL HELP

For some of us, professional help, such as therapy or counseling, may be the most appropriate form of support. Grief counselors and therapists are trained to provide evidence-based interventions and strategies for managing the complex emotions and challenges of grief. They can offer a safe and confidential haven to process emotions, develop coping skills, and address any related mental health concerns, such as depression or anxiety.

SUPPORT GROUPS

Support groups can invite their own form of healing. Rather than grieving in isolation, we might find from a support group a sense of community by connecting with others who have experienced similar losses. Some groups are led by trained facilitators. Other equally effective groups can be peer-supported. While general support can be helpful, some of us might benefit more from a group that focuses on specific types of loss, such as the death of a spouse or child. In support groups we can learn from others and share our experiences when we're ready. At any stage, we may feel less alone in the grieving process.

ONLINE SUPPORT

In today's digital age, online support has become an increasingly popular and accessible option if we're grieving. Online support can take many forms, from social media groups to forums to virtual support groups. These platforms can be a lifeline, especially for those of us who are physically isolated or unable to access in-person support. Unlike face-to-face support, virtual communication has potential drawbacks. Two important concerns worth noting are a potential lack of privacy and a greater possibility for receiving misinformation.

MENTORING

Mentoring, which we will discuss in more detail later, can be a particularly powerful form of support when we're grieving. Unlike professional help or support groups, mentoring invites a one-on-one relationship built on trust and empathy. Mentoring can be especially dynamic if the mentor and mentee have common grief experiences. Through practical advice based on their own experiences of loss, mentors guide and support mentees. Early results include helping the mentees feel less alone and more equipped to navigate the challenges of grief.

SELF-CARE

While seeking external support is important, it is also crucial to prioritize self-care during the grieving process. Self-care can take many forms, from engaging in activities that bring joy and relaxation to maintaining a healthy lifestyle through exercise and nutrition.

Seeking support during the grieving process will look different for each of us. Different types of support can be beneficial at various stages of the journey. What works for one person may not work for another. For instance, professional help, such as counseling or therapy, can be particularly useful in the early stages of grief, when emotions are raw and overwhelming. A trained mental health professional may open a safe space to process these emotions and develop coping strategies. As the grieving process progresses, support groups and mentoring relationships can help us build community and connection so that we feel less alone.

In my own journey, a combination of professional help, peer support, and mentoring has been instrumental in working my way through the complexities of grief. Initially, I was hesitant to reach out for help, believing that I could handle everything on my own. However, when I finally accepted the support that was offered, I gleened immense value from sharing my experiences and emotions with others who understood what I was going through. The guidance and wisdom of a counselor, coupled with the empathy and understanding of peers in a support group, helped me process my grief in a healthy way. As a mentor, I now strive to offer that same level of support and understanding to others who are struggling. I can sense my guidance and perspective making a positive impact, especially when I draw from my own experiences with grief.

Ultimately, the most empowering perspective is being open to seeking and accepting support in whatever form feels most comfortable and beneficial to you. It may require stepping out of your comfort zone and being vulnerable with others. But the rewards—in terms of emotional healing, personal growth, and a sense of connection—can be immeasurable. Embracing a range of support options can create a comprehensive support network.

EXERCISE PATIENCE AND SELF-COMPASSION

Approach the grieving process with patience and self-compassion. Recognize that healing takes time. Setbacks and challenges are a normal part of the experience. Grief is a journey of ups and downs. Avoid pressuring yourself to heal in a specific time frame. Instead, practice patience.

Rather than judging yourself, nurture yourself with compassion. Only then can you express the full range of emotions that come with loss, without judgment or criticism. Treat yourself with kindness and understanding. When necessary, forgive yourself. In so doing, you will make your environment one of profound healing.

Self-compassion develops in many forms. Three simple, self-generated practices can result in significant gains.

ACKNOWLEDGE AND VALIDATE YOUR EMOTIONS

Rather than trying to suppress or ignore difficult emotions, acknowledge them. Even if they feel strange and unlike you, validate them. A simple start can be simply recognizing that feelings of sadness, anger, and despair are normal and understandable responses to loss.

Practice Self-Care

An essential component of compassion, self-care entails taking steps to nurture and support yourself during difficult times. Self-care takes many different forms. You can engage in activities that bring you joy or help you feel relaxed. You might set boundaries for your time and energy. You could seek support when needed.

Challenge Self-Critical Thoughts

Self-critical thoughts often accompany grief. We might tell ourselves, "I should be handling this better" or "I'm not grieving the right way." Challenge these thoughts. Further, replace them with more compassionate and understanding messages, such as "I am doing the best I can" or "There is no right or wrong way to grieve."

Seeking support is a crucial component of navigating the grieving process and promoting mental health and well-being. Whether through professional help, support groups, mentoring relationships, or self-care practices, finding the right support can help you feel less alone, more understood, and better equipped to manage the challenges of grief.

Ultimately, the key to seeking support during the grieving process is to approach the journey with patience, self-compassion, and a willingness to reach out for help when needed. Sometimes, a combination of different types of support might help you most. At other times, different forms of support can feel most appropriate at different stages of grieving. Beyond the inner work you do to heal, invite support from outsides sources whose help can be both profound and meaningful.

CHAPTER 6

GRIEF MENTORING

MENTORING IS A PROFOUND RELATIONSHIP that entails the exchange of knowledge, experience, and insights between two individuals, typically involving someone who may be more experienced, known as the mentor, and another who is less experienced, referred to as the mentee or protégé. This relationship plays a pivotal role in the personal and professional development of the mentee. In some cases, it also benefits the mentor.

Mentoring relationships can extend beyond traditional career or academic contexts and provide invaluable support in navigating life's most challenging experiences, including grief and loss. The wisdom, empathy, and guidance offered by a mentor who has walked a similar path can be a lifeline for individuals struggling to cope with the profound emotional and practical implications of bereavement.

Grief mentoring is a form of mentorship specifically focused on providing guidance, support, and companionship to individuals who are grieving the loss of a loved one. It involves an experienced mentor, someone who has gone through their own profound grief journey, coming alongside a mentee to help them navigate the complex and often disorienting emotions, challenges, and life transitions that accompany bereavement.

At its core, grief mentoring recognizes that while grief is an inevitable part of the human experience, it can also be an extraordinarily lonely and overwhelming process. A grief mentor serves as a compassionate, non-judgmental presence who can bear witness to the mentee's pain through empathetic listening and sharing their own hard-won insights and coping strategies.

Let's delve deeper into various aspects of mentoring and how it can be a helpful form of support for navigating grief.

TYPES OF MENTORING

There are different types of mentoring. While they all share similarities, each also offers some unique support.

TRADITIONAL ONE-ON-ONE MENTORING

In this most common type of mentoring, an experienced individual (mentor) is paired with a less experienced individual (mentee) to provide guidance, support, and advice. Based on their experience, the mentor shares their knowledge and skills to help the mentee grow personally or professionally. This type of mentoring is often used in academic and workplace settings but is not limited to these settings. In the context of grief mentoring, this approach can involve an experienced individual who has navigated the grieving process themselves providing one-on-one guidance and support to someone currently dealing with loss and bereavement.

GROUP MENTORING

In this type of mentoring, one mentor works with a small group of mentees simultaneously. The mentor facilitates discussions to the group as a whole. In this context, mentors share experiences and provide guidance. Besides learning from the mentor, mentees learn from each other's experiences and perspectives, fostering a sense of community and collaboration. This type of mentoring is often used in educational and training programs. For those grieving, group mentoring can create a supportive community where individuals can share their experiences, learn from others on similar journeys, and receive collective wisdom from a mentor who has overcome grief.

PEER MENTORING

Peer mentoring involves individuals at similar levels of experience or expertise mentoring each other. This type of mentoring is based on the idea that individuals can learn from each other's experiences and provide mutual support. Peer mentoring is often used in academic settings, such as universities or schools, where students mentor each other. Peer mentoring can be particularly powerful for grief support, as individuals at similar stages of the grieving process can share coping strategies, validate each other's emotions, and provide mutual understanding.

REVERSE MENTORING

Reverse mentoring flips the traditional mentoring model, with a younger or less experienced individual mentoring an older or more experienced individual. This type of mentoring is often used to help senior executives stay current with new technologies, trends, or perspectives. It can also foster cross-generational understanding and collaboration. In terms of grief, reverse mentoring could involve a younger person who has experienced a significant loss mentoring an older individual, fostering cross-generational understanding and new perspectives on the grieving experience.

E-MENTORING OR VIRTUAL MENTORING

E-mentoring, also known as virtual mentoring, involves using electronic communication tools, such as email, video conferencing, or online platforms, to facilitate mentoring relationships. This type of mentoring allows mentors and mentees to connect regardless of geographic location or time constraints. E-mentoring is particularly useful for connecting individuals across different offices, countries, or time zones.

Virtual grief mentoring can bridge geographical barriers, allowing individuals to connect with mentors who have navigated loss, regardless of their location, providing accessible support during a time of immense emotional challenges.

Situational Mentoring

Situational mentoring is a short-term, targeted form of mentoring that focuses on helping the mentee navigate a specific challenge or situation. The mentor provides guidance and support to help the mentee develop the skills and strategies needed to address the specific issue at hand. This type of mentoring is often used in the workplace to help employees through career transitions, new projects, or specific skill development. For those facing specific challenges related to grief, such as facing the loss of a spouse or child, or planning end-of-life arrangements, situational mentors with relevant experiences can offer targeted guidance to help mentees through these difficult situations.

Mentoring Circles

Mentoring circles involve a group of individuals who come together to support and learn from each other. Each member of the circle takes turns being the mentor, sharing their experiences and expertise with the group. This type of mentoring fosters a sense of community and allows individuals to build a diverse network of support. Mentoring circles are often used in professional development and leadership training programs. Grief mentoring circles can create a sense of community and mutual understanding, with members taking turns sharing their journeys and supporting one another through the various stages and complexities of the grieving process.

Informal Mentoring

Informal mentoring relationships develop naturally, without a formal structure or program. These relationships often arise when an experienced individual takes an interest in supporting and guiding a less experienced individual. Informal mentoring can occur in various settings, such as the workplace, community organizations, or personal networks. Informal grief mentoring relationships can develop organically, often initiated by someone seeking guidance and support from an individual they know has successfully navigated the grieving process, providing a more personal and relatable connection.

FLASH MENTORING

Flash mentoring is a brief, one-time mentoring session that focuses on a specific topic or question. This type of mentoring is often used at events or conferences, where attendees can sign up for short mentoring sessions with experienced professionals. Flash mentoring allows individuals to gain quick insights and advice on specific topics or challenges. At events or gatherings related to grief and loss, flash mentoring sessions can provide individuals with the opportunity to gain quick insights and advice from experienced grief mentors on specific challenges or questions they may have.

DIVERSITY MENTORING

Diversity mentoring focuses on supporting individuals from underrepresented or diverse backgrounds, such as women or minorities. The mentor, who may or may not be from the same background as the mentee, provides guidance and support to help the mentee overcome challenges specific to their identity or experience. Diversity mentoring aims to foster inclusion, equity, and diversity in various settings, such as the workplace or educational institutions. For individuals from diverse backgrounds, grief mentoring can be tailored to address the unique cultural, religious, or identity-related aspects that may influence their grieving experiences, ensuring a more inclusive and respectful support system.

While there are many different approaches to mentoring, what remains constant is the power of having a supportive guide who can provide empathic wisdom drawn from their own experiences with grief and loss. Whether it's the intimacy of one-on-one mentoring, the community found in group or peer mentoring circles, or the tailored guidance of situational mentors, each modality offers a path toward healing.

In the end, the most effective grief mentoring allows the mentor to attune to the unique needs of the mentee based on where they are in their journey. Sometimes that may call for the compassionate listening ear of an informal mentor. Other times, it could be the logistical expertise of someone who has navigated specific challenges like the loss of a spouse or child.

What remains universal is the power of human connection to help illumine the way through the darkness of grief. By sharing their hard-won perspectives while still honoring each person's individual process, grief mentors can be beacons of hope. Their guidance provides handrails for mentees to move through the gnawing emptiness and disorientation of profound loss.

While no mentor can undo the pain of bereavement, their role is to compassionately bear witness, offer coping strategies, and help the grieving person integrate their loss into a new norm where growth and meaning can eventually take root once more. The path is arduous, but skilled mentors can light the way toward the other side of sorrow.

COMPONENTS OF A MENTORING RELATIONSHIP

Effective mentoring relationships consist of several key components that contribute to their success and mutual benefit. Here are the essential components of a mentoring relationship.

TRUST AND RESPECT

A strong foundation of trust and respect is crucial for a successful mentoring relationship. Both the mentor and the mentee must establish an environment of mutual trust, where they can openly share their thoughts, concerns, and vulnerabilities without fear of judgement or repercussions. Respect for each other's perspectives, experiences, and boundaries is essential for fostering a healthy and productive relationship.

CLEAR EXPECTATIONS AND GOALS

At the outset of the mentoring relationship, it is important to establish clear expectations and goals. Together, the mentor and mentee should align their objectives. Through a clear discussion of their respective roles and responsibilities, they can also set realistic timelines for achieving specific goals. This clarity helps to ensure that both parties are working towards the same desired outcomes and minimizes potential misunderstandings or disappointments.

OPEN AND HONEST COMMUNICATION

Effective communication is the lifeblood of a mentoring relationship. Both the mentor and the mentee should cultivate an environment of transparent communication where they feel free to be open and honest. Meaningful discussions require active listening and providing constructive feedback. The result is a helpful exchange of ideas, insights, and perspectives. Regular check-ins and progress updates are also essential for maintaining open lines of communication.

COMMITMENT AND DEDICATION

A successful mentoring relationship requires a committed investment of time and effort from both parties. The mentor must be dedicated to sharing their knowledge and experience, while the mentee must be committed to actively listening, learning, and implementing the guidance provided. Consistent engagement and follow-through on agreed-upon actions are crucial for sustaining the momentum and achieving desired outcomes.

CONFIDENTIALITY AND TRUST

Confidentiality is a critical component of a mentoring relationship, as it fosters an environment of trust and openness.

Both parties should agree to maintain confidentiality regarding sensitive information shared during their interactions, unless explicitly agreed upon otherwise. This sense of privacy and trust allows for more vulnerable and authentic conversations, leading to better results.

Constructive Feedback and Accountability

Mentors play a vital role in providing constructive feedback to their mentees. This feedback should be delivered in a supportive and empathetic manner, focusing on areas for improvement and offering practical suggestions for growth. At the same time, mentees should be accountable for their actions and receptive to feedback, demonstrating a willingness to implement the guidance provided.

Empowerment and Encouragement

An effective mentor empowers and encourages their mentee to develop skills and reach their full potential as they pursue their goals. Beyond providing emotional support, the mentor helps boost the mentee's confidence and celebrates their successes along the way. In this way, the mentor serves as a source of motivation and inspiration, helping the mentee overcome challenges and embrace new opportunities for growth.

Continuous Learning and Adaptation

Mentoring establishes dynamic, evolving relationships that require both parties to engage in continuous learning and adaptation. As the mentee progresses and their needs change, the mentor should be flexible in their approach, continually tailoring their guidance to meet the mentee's evolving goals and circumstances.

When these components are present, mentoring relationships can foster a supportive, nurturing environment that meets its purpose for both mentor and mentee. It is a transformative experience that can have a lasting impact on individuals' lives that contributes to their overall success and fulfillment.

In the context of grief, mentoring relationships can play a crucial role in providing guidance and support. Mentors create a safe space for the mentee to explore the complex emotions and challenges that come with loss. With empathy, a mentor who has experienced similar grief can offer invaluable wisdom and suggest practical strategies for coping and healing. Conversely, mentees can find solace and build emotional strength by sharing their experiences with someone who truly understands their pain.

The trust, open communication, and confidentiality inherent in a healthy mentoring relationship can create an environment where individuals can freely express their grief without fear of judgment. When mentors offer constructive feedback while expecting accountability, they help mentees process their emotions in a healthy manner that develops resilience. A mentor's encouragement can empower mentees to honor their grief as they find the courage to embrace new possibilities for growth and healing.

WHAT MENTORING INVOLVES

As a grief mentor, I find that more and more people grappling with profound loss are reaching out for the support they need to begin and continue on their healing journey. But what does grief mentoring truly entail? It can involve a range of activities aimed at providing compassionate guidance. Grief mentors may:

SHARE PERSPECTIVES ON GRIEF

A mentor's lived experience with grief is an invaluable resource for the mentee. Sharing personal insights gives mentors the opportunity to impart hard-won wisdom that can help illuminate the mentee's own path through bereavement. While sharing profound perspectives, it is appropriate for a mentor to do the following:

Offer Personal Grief Narratives

The mentor may recount their own transformative experiences and the journey they took through loss. These intimate narratives contain powerful lessons the mentee can absorb without having to endure the same suffering firsthand.

Process Emotions

In addition to stories, mentors can share insights into the vast emotional landscape of grief—making sense of complicated feelings like guilt, anger, yearning, and eventual acceptance. Throughout this emotional journey, mentors may:

Model Coping Strategies

By learning about the mentor's own coping mechanisms and what brought them solace, the mentee can gain a toolkit of potential strategies as they chart their own course.

Validate Feelings

A mentor helps the mentee explore a vast array of feelings. Sadness and anger and guilt are only a few. During this exploration, mentors can help mentees understand any emotion is normal and permissible as part of the grieving process.

Reframe Perspectives

When the mentee is stuck in patterns of negativity or self-blame, the mentor can compassionately reframe perspectives based on their own hard-won wisdom.

Suggest Coping Tools

Mentors provide an experienced vantage point to evaluate the mentee's coping mechanisms. With care, they can recommend alternative tools like journaling, rituals, or support groups.

OFFER EMPATHY AND ENCOURAGEMENT

In addition to practical advice, a grief mentor can be a vital source of empathy, emotional reassurance and motivation when the journey feels insurmountable. A good mentor will:

LISTEN EMPATHICALLY

A mentor can be a compassionate sounding board, allowing the mentee to express the depths of their pain and emotions without judgement.

FOSTER RESILIENCE

When mentees feel depleted, mentors can help them reconnect with their own inner reserves of strength and perseverance that enabled survival thus far.

CELEBRATE MILESTONES

By gently honoring incremental steps like getting through challenges, mentors can instill confidence and resilience in the mentee's ability to evolve through grief.

FACILITATE HEALING CONNECTIONS

One of the mentor's greatest gifts is the opportunity to facilitate connections that can aid the healing process. To do so, they may:

SHARE STORIES

By being vulnerable with their own experiences, the mentor normalizes grieving and losing isolation. Story sharing creates a bonding experience.

BUILD COMMUNITY

Grief mentors can recommend or facilitate mentee involvement in support groups, inviting connections with others on similar paths.

Access Resources

With their own lived experience, mentors can guide mentees toward helpful books, therapists, rituals, and other healing resources.

DYNAMICS OF A MENTORING RELATIONSHIP

The dynamics that govern a mentoring relationship play a pivotal role in determining its effectiveness and longevity. These dynamics encompass various factors, including the nature of the relationship itself, the shared values and mindsets of the mentor and mentee, and the mutual commitment to the mentoring process. Understanding and nurturing these dynamics is essential for cultivating a productive, rewarding mentoring experience.

Formal or Informal

One of the fundamental dynamics to consider is whether the mentoring relationship is formal or informal.

Formal mentoring relationships are often structured and facilitated through organized programs within organizations or educational institutions. These relationships typically have defined goals, timelines, and expectations, with regular check-ins and evaluations.

Informal mentoring relationships tend to develop organically, often initiated by the mentee's admiration for the mentor's expertise or personal qualities. These relationships may be more fluid and adaptable, allowing for a more natural rapport and tailored approach.

Respect and Trust

Regardless of the formality or informality of the relationship, mutual respect and trust are paramount. The mentee must value and respect the mentor's wisdom, experience, and guidance, acknowledging their authority and credibility in the respective domain. Conversely, the mentor must respect the mentee's ambitions, ideas, and perspectives, recognizing their potential for growth and development. This mutual respect and trust create an environment of psychological safety, where both parties feel comfortable expressing their thoughts, concerns, and vulnerabilities without fear of judgment or repercussions.

GROWTH AND LEARNING

Moreover, a shared commitment to growth and learning is a critical dynamic that underpins a successful mentoring relationship. Both the mentor and mentee must approach the relationship with a genuine desire to learn, develop, and expand their knowledge and capabilities. The mentor should be driven by a passion for sharing their expertise and contributing to the mentee's growth, while the mentee should be eager to absorb the mentor's insights and apply them to their perceived development.

COMMUNICATION AND UNDERSTANDING

Effective communication is essential. Both parties should strive to understand and adapt to each other's communication preferences. Whether it's direct or more nuanced, only clear communication can facilitate open and productive dialogue.

GOALS AND EXPECTATIONS

At the outset of the mentoring relationship, it is crucial to align goals to ensure that both parties are working towards common objectives. Further, the mentor and mentee should establish clear expectations so they can measure progress effectively.

FLEXIBILITY AND ADAPTABILITY

As mentoring relationships evolve, both the mentor and mentee should exhibit flexibility and adaptability. Commonly, progress in the relationship will require them both to adjust their approaches and strategies as needed to accommodate changing circumstances or evolving needs.

BENEFITS FOR MENTEES

Mentoring relationships can be incredibly beneficial for individuals navigating the complex, often overwhelming experience of grief. By providing a supportive and understanding environment, mentors and mentees can find solace, growth, and healing through their shared journey.

Throughout and as a result of their mentorship relationship, mentees can expect to gain many benefits.

EMOTIONAL SUPPORT AND EMPATHY

Grieving individuals often feel misunderstood and alone in their pain. A mentor who has walked a similar path can offer a compassionate ear and a deep sense of empathy, validating the mentee's emotions and helping them feel less isolated in their grief. This understanding can be a profound source of comfort and healing.

COPING STRATEGIES AND RESILIENCE

Mentors often share their personal experiences and describe the coping strategies they utilized to navigate the challenges of grief. By learning from their mentor's wisdom, mentees can develop a toolbox of healthy coping mechanisms. These may include practicing mindfulness, journaling, or engaging in meaningful activities. Such strategies can help mentees cultivate resilience, enabling them to navigate the ebbs and flows of grief with greater ease.

PERSONAL GROWTH AND SELF-DISCOVERY

Grief can be a transformative experience, prompting individuals to reassess their values, beliefs, and even their purpose in life. A mentor can guide the mentee through this process of self-discovery, offering a safe space to explore existential questions and uncover newfound strength and meaning. This personal growth can lead to a deeper understanding of oneself and a renewed appreciation for life's journey.

INSPIRATION AND HOPE

Witnessing a mentor's ability to heal and find meaning after loss can be a powerful source of inspiration and hope for the mentee. The mentor's journey serves as a living example that it is possible to emerge from the depths of grief and embrace a fulfilling life once again. This inspiration can fuel the mentee's determination and provide the courage to move forward.

BENEFITS FOR MENTORS

While mentorship relationships are formed for the purpose of helping the mentee, its benefits to the mentor can also be profound. Thanks to such relationships, mentors gain or build on rich qualities that add meaning to life.

PURPOSE AND LEGACY

By sharing their experiences and wisdom with a mentee, mentors can find a profound sense of purpose and leave a lasting legacy. Knowing that their guidance has positively impacted someone's healing journey can be immensely rewarding. That fulfillment invokes a sense of contribution that can feel profoundly meaningful.

PERSONAL GROWTH AND SELF-REFLECTION

The process of mentoring often prompts mentors to revisit their own grief journey. In the process they often gain new insights and perspectives. This self-reflection can lead to personal growth, a deeper understanding of their own experiences with loss, and the potential to continue their own healing process.

Giving Back and Paying it Forward

For many, the act of mentoring is a way to give back and pay forward the support they received during their own time of need. It allows them to honor the memory of their loved ones and create a ripple effect of healing and compassion, ensuring that their experiences can positively impact others.

Community and Belonging

Mentoring relationships can forge deep connections between individuals who share the common bond of grief. These connections can provide a sense of community and belonging. They remind both mentors and mentees that they are not alone in their journeys. This shared understanding can foster a powerful sense of kinship in the context of mutual support.

Continued Healing and Growth

For mentors, the process of sharing their experiences can be cathartic. As they reflect on their grief journey, they also witness the mentee's progress. This dual perspective may give mentors newfound insights. Through them, mentors often resolve lingering aspects of their own grief. Finding such closure can be empowering.

Whether mentors or mentees, individuals involved in mentoring relationships within the context of grief can experience profound personal and emotional growth, healing, and transformation. Mentoring can, therefore, serve as a catalyst for self-discovery, resilience, and the cultivation of meaning and purpose in the face of life's most challenging experiences.

While deeply rewarding, mentoring relationships can also present various challenges, particularly in the context of grief mentoring. Mentees, as well was their mentors, may face unique obstacles throughout the complex and emotionally charged terrain of loss and healing.

CHALLENGES FOR MENTEES

Even mentees eager to secure this kind of support will likely encounter emotional challenges throughout the process.

TRUST AND VULNERABILITY

Opening up about the deeply personal and emotional experience of grief requires a significant level of trust and vulnerability. Fearing judgment or misunderstanding, mentees may struggle to fully disclose their thoughts, feelings, and challenges.

EMOTIONAL DEPENDENCE

While emotional support is a crucial aspect of grief mentoring, mentees may inadvertently develop an unhealthy emotional dependence on their mentors. This can hinder their ability to develop their own coping mechanisms and resilience, ultimately impeding their healing process.

RESISTANCE OR AVOIDANCE

Grief can be an overwhelming and painful experience. Mentees may resist confronting their pain or avoid processing their emotions. Either diverting strategy can create barriers in the mentoring relationship and impede progress.

UNREALISTIC EXPECTATIONS

Mentees may hold unrealistic expectations about the mentoring relationship or the mentor's ability to "fix" their grief. When these expectations are not met, it can lead to disappointment and frustration. In some cases, it can completely break down the mentoring dynamic.

CHALLENGES FOR MENTORS

Even seasoned mentors need to remain cognizant of unique challenges their role presents.

VULNERABILITY

Sharing personal experiences related to grief can be emotionally taxing for mentors. Revisiting painful memories and emotions may trigger unresolved grief or reopen old wounds, leading to feelings of vulnerability and potential emotional exhaustion.

BOUNDARIES

Mentors must strike a delicate balance between feeling empathy and maintaining appropriate boundaries. While cultivating a supportive and understanding relationship is crucial, mentors may struggle to establish healthy boundaries, risking emotional over-involvement or vicarious trauma.

Vicarious trauma refers to the emotional distress and trauma-like symptoms that can arise in those who are repeatedly exposed to the firsthand trauma experiences of others. For grief mentors who are consistently holding space for mentees' stories of profound loss and pain, there is a risk of internalizing some of that suffering over time. This can lead to symptoms similar to post-traumatic stress, such as intrusive thoughts, avoidance behaviors, hypervigilance, and even physical manifestations like chronic exhaustion or illness. Establishing clear boundaries around how much of the mentee's traumatic grief they can take on while still maintaining their own equilibrium is essential for mentors to avoid this form of secondary traumatic stress.

OBJECTIVITY

Despite their own experiences with grief, mentors must strive to maintain objectivity and impartiality when guiding their mentees. Indulging personal biases or projecting their own grief journey onto the mentee's experiences can hinder effective mentoring and lead to misunderstandings or misguided advice.

EXPECTATIONS

Grief is a highly personal and complex experience. Every individual's journey is unique. Mentors may face the challenge of managing their mentees' expectations. Personally, mentors must recognize that their guidance and support can only go so far. Ultimately, each person must find their own path to healing.

The power of mentoring relationships lies in the mentor's ability to provide a supportive and compassionate environment where mentees can embark on a transformative journey that cultivates resilience and self-discovery. For both parties to honor the profound lessons that grief can teach us, they must foster open communication, mutual respect, and a shared commitment to growth. While challenges may arise, the mentoring experience in the context of grief has the potential to create a profound and lasting impact. Ultimately, it can leave both mentors and mentees with a renewed sense of purpose, connection, and the strength to embrace life's continual unfolding with grace and wisdom.

CHAPTER 7

MENTORS AS BRIDGES TO MENTAL HEALTH SUPPORT

WE LIVE IN AN ERA of rising mental health challenges. Grief and loss are having a profound impact on individuals as well as entire communities. Ensuring access to comprehensive and effective support systems has become a pressing priority. While professional mental health services play a crucial role in addressing these issues, significant barriers often hinder individuals from seeking or accessing the care they need.

Financial constraints, geographic limitations, cultural stigma, and a shortage of qualified mental health professionals are just a few of the obstacles that can create gaps in the mental health care continuum. These gaps can leave individuals feeling isolated, overwhelmed, and without the resources necessary to navigate the complexities of grief and its impact on their mental well-being.

Within this landscape mentors emerge as invaluable bridges, connecting individuals in need with the support and guidance they require. Mentors, drawing from their own lived experiences and a deep well of empathy, can provide a compassionate presence and a safe space for mentees to express their emotions, share their stories, and begin the process of healing and growth.

Mentors play an essential role in bridging the gap between individuals and professional mental health support, particularly in the context of grief and its impact on mental health. By serving as guides, connectors, and advocates, mentors can help mentees navigate the often-complex mental health system. In this role they can also help mentees identify appropriate resources and ultimately foster a more comprehensive and holistic approach to mental well-being.

THE UNMET NEED FOR MENTAL HEALTH SERVICES

The world is grappling with a burgeoning mental health crisis that has far-reaching implications for individuals, communities, and societies as a whole. According to the World Health Organization, nearly one billion people globally are living with a mental disorder, a staggering figure that underscores the urgency of addressing this pressing issue. Mental health conditions can manifest in various forms, ranging from depression and anxiety to more severe disorders, such as schizophrenia and bipolar disorder.

In its wake, the COVID-19 pandemic further exacerbated the mental health crisis. Increased rates of stress, isolation, and grief took a toll on the psychological well-being of individuals worldwide. The disruption of daily routines, loss of loved ones, and economic uncertainties contributed to a surge in mental health challenges, highlighting the need for comprehensive and accessible support systems.

Even before the COVID-19 pandemic, other barriers to accessing professional mental health treatment existed. Despite the growing recognition of mental health as a critical public health concern, significant barriers persist in accessing professional treatment and support services. Financial constraints, lack of insurance coverage, and the high cost of mental health care can make it prohibitively expensive for many individuals, particularly those from low-income or marginalized communities.

Geographic limitations also pose a significant challenge, with rural and remote areas often facing a shortage of qualified mental health professionals or specialized treatment facilities. In urban areas, long waiting lists and limited availability of providers can create further obstacles to timely and adequate care.

Cultural stigma and societal attitudes towards mental health also play a role in deterring individuals from seeking professional help. The pervasive stigma surrounding mental illness can lead to feelings of shame, fear of discrimination, and a reluctance to acknowledge or address mental health concerns, further perpetuating the cycle of unmet needs.

Early intervention and accessible support are crucial to addressing mental health concerns before they escalate into more severe and challenging conditions. Untreated mental health issues can have far-reaching consequences, including decreased productivity, strained relationships, substance abuse, and in some cases, self-harm or suicide.

By providing early intervention and support, individuals can develop coping mechanisms, access appropriate resources, and receive guidance and treatment before their mental health deteriorates further. Early intervention can also help prevent the onset of more severe mental health conditions and promote overall well-being and resilience.

In the context of grief and loss, early support can be particularly important in mitigating the mental health impacts of traumatic experiences and helping individuals navigate the complex emotions and challenges that often accompany bereavement.

THE VALUE OF MENTORSHIP IN GRIEF AND MENTAL HEALTH

Mentors play a vital role in creating a safe and supportive environment for individuals navigating the complex interplay of grief and mental health. With the cultivation of a compassionate and non-judgmental space provided by mentors, mentees feel free to express their thoughts, feelings, and experiences without fear of stigma or discrimination.

In the aftermath of loss, individuals may grapple with a wide range of emotions, including sadness, anger, guilt, and anxiety. A mentor's ability to actively listen, validate these feelings, and offer a non-judgmental presence can provide immense comfort and support during this difficult time.

Through active listening and thoughtful questioning, mentors can encourage mentees to share their experiences, fears, and challenges related to grief and mental health. This open dialogue not only helps mentors better understand the mentee's unique circumstances but also allows mentees to process their emotions and gain valuable insights and perspectives.

While mentors are not meant to replace professional mental health services, they can provide initial emotional support and guidance to mentees as they navigate the complexities of grief and its impact on their mental well-being.

Mentors can offer a compassionate ear, validate the mentee's emotions, and share their own experiences and insights related to grief and loss. They can also introduce coping strategies to help mentees develop healthy coping mechanisms and promote resilience.

By providing this initial emotional support and guidance, mentors can serve as a crucial first line of defense, helping mentees process their emotions and identify when professional mental health services may be needed.

MENTORS AS GUIDES AND CONNECTORS

While mentors can offer invaluable emotional support and guidance, it is crucial for them to recognize the limitations of their role and the importance of seeking professional help when needed. With proper training and awareness, mentors can learn to identify signs and symptoms that may indicate the need for more specialized mental health intervention.

For example, mentors should be attuned to indicators such as persistent and overwhelming sadness, hopelessness, or suicidal ideation. These may signify the presence of more severe mental health conditions like major depressive disorder or post-traumatic stress disorder (PTSD). In such cases, a good mentor can play a vital role in encouraging and facilitating mentee's access to professional mental health services, if needed.

The mental health system can be complex and overwhelming to navigate, particularly for those unfamiliar with the available resources or unsure of where to begin searching for support. Mentors can serve as knowledgeable guides, helping mentees understand the various options and select the most helpful services available.

Mentors may provide information on local mental health clinics, counseling centers, support groups, or specialized treatment facilities. Mentors can also assist mentees in understanding the different levels of care, such as outpatient therapy, intensive outpatient programs, or inpatient treatment. Finally, they can help them determine the most appropriate course of action based on their specific needs and circumstances.

While recognizing the need for professional help is a crucial first step, the process of actively seeking out and accessing mental health services can be daunting for many individuals. Mentors can play a vital role in encouraging mentees throughout this process.

Mentors can support in various ways. They may need to validate the importance of seeking help. They may be called upon to address the stigma or fears related to mental health treatment. They may recognize a mentee's need of emotional support and encouragement throughout the journey.

Simple tasks can seem overwhelming to mentees in the throes of grief. At such times, mentors can also provide practical assistance. Explaining insurance coverage, scheduling appointments, or identifying transportation options to ensure access to care could make possible for mentees what feels insurmountable.

By fostering a supportive and non-judgmental environment, mentors can empower mentees to take proactive steps towards their mental health and well-being. Such help ultimately facilitates a smoother transition to professional care and support.

COLLABORATION BETWEEN MENTORS AND MENTAL HEALTH PROFESSIONALS

While mentors can serve as valuable initial sources of support and guidance, it is crucial to recognize the limitations of their role and the importance of collaboration with mental health professionals. By establishing partnerships and referral systems, mentors can ensure a seamless transition for mentees to receive specialized care and treatment from qualified professionals.

These partnerships may require regular communication and information-sharing between mentors and mental health professionals. Such coordinated approaches effectively support the mentee's mental health journey. Communication can work from either direction. Mental health professionals may provide mentors with guidance on appropriate responses, boundaries, and strategies for supporting mentees, while mentors can offer valuable insights into the mentee's personal experiences and unique needs.

Collaboration between mentors and mental health professionals can also involve sharing insights and perspectives that creates a continuum of care to address the multifaceted needs of mentees. While mental health professionals provide mentors with clinical insights and evidence-based practices, mentors can offer firsthand accounts of the lived experiences of grief and mental health challenges.

By fostering open communication and sharing insights, mentors and mental health professionals can work together to develop comprehensive support plans tailored to the mentee's emotional, psychological, and practical needs. This collaborative approach ensures that mentees receive holistic care and support, with mentors and professionals each contributing their unique expertise and perspectives.

Mentors can also play a crucial role in addressing the stigma surrounding mental health and promoting awareness within their communities. By openly discussing their experiences and the value of seeking professional support, mentors can help normalize conversations around mental health and encourage others to prioritize their well-being.

Through their partnerships with mental health professionals, mentors can receive guidance and resources to facilitate educational outreach and awareness campaigns. These efforts can help dispel myths, challenge stereotypes, and promote a deeper understanding of mental health as a critical aspect of overall well-being.

These efforts can contribute to creating a more inclusive and supportive environment for individuals in grief. Improved access to care helps foster a culture of compassion and understanding.

MENTOR CAPACITY AND COMPETENCY

To effectively support mentees through mental health challenges like grief, competent mentors must possess a robust set of skills. Training on active listening techniques is essential, as it enables mentors to fully engage with mentees, validate their experiences, and create a safe, non-judgmental space for open communication.

Moreover, mentors should receive training in crisis intervention that equips them with the knowledge to recognize and the skill to respond appropriately to mental health emergencies or situations of heightened risk. This training can include identifying warning signs, implementing de-escalation strategies, and understanding when and how to involve professional support or emergency services.

Setting and maintaining appropriate boundaries is another critical aspect of mentor training. Good mentors understand the limitations of their role. They value the importance of establishing healthy boundaries to protect both themselves and their mentees. This includes recognizing situations that may require referral to professional mental health services. Mentors appropriately walk the delicate tightrope between providing support and avoiding over-involvement or enabling unhealthy dependencies.

In addition to practical skills, mentors must develop a comprehensive understanding of various mental health conditions, their symptoms, and appropriate responses. Being able to recognize potential mental health concerns early, mentors can provide appropriate guidance and support to their mentees.

Training should cover a range of mental health conditions, including depression, anxiety disorders, PTSD, and grief-related disorders, among others. Mentors should learn about the unique challenges and manifestations of each condition, as well as evidence-based coping strategies and self-care practices that can be shared with mentees.

Mentors must also cultivate cultural competence. They should adopt trauma-informed approaches that provide sensitive, tailored support to mentees from diverse backgrounds and with varying experiences of trauma or adversity. Cultural competence involves developing an understanding and appreciation of different cultural beliefs, values, and practices surrounding mental health and grief.

Trauma-informed approaches, on the other hand, recognize the prevalence and impact of trauma. They incorporate principles such as safety, choice, collaboration, and empowerment into the mentoring relationship. This equips mentors with the ability to create a more inclusive and supportive environment that acknowledges and responds to the unique needs and experiences of each mentee.

MENTORSHIP IN COMMUNITY MENTAL HEALTH INITIATIVES

To truly leverage the power of mentorship in addressing mental health needs, it is essential to integrate mentors into broader community mental health initiatives. Collaborating with local organizations, support groups, and mental health advocacy efforts enables mentors to serve as valuable community resources while advocating for mental health awareness and support.

Mentors can play a pivotal role in outreach and education efforts. By sharing their experience-based insights, they help destigmatize mental health conversations. Even more powerfully, they encourage help-seeking behaviors within their communities. In this way they can serve as ambassadors, connecting individuals in need with available mental health resources. They play an essential role in ensuring no one faces their struggles alone.

Collaboration with local organizations and support groups is crucial for creating a comprehensive, coordinated approach to mental health support. Mentors can partner with community-based organizations, religious institutions, schools, and mental health advocacy groups to identify areas of need and develop targeted initiatives to address them.

By working closely with these organizations, mentors can gain access to additional resources, training opportunities, and referral networks, further enhancing their ability to provide effective support to mentees. Additionally, mentors can contribute their unique perspectives to inform the development and implementation of community-based mental health services.

The integration of mentorship into community mental health initiatives should aim to create a supportive network that fosters mental health and well-being for all members of the community. This network should encompass mentors, mental health professionals, community organizations, and local resources, working in tandem to provide a continuum of care and support.

Within this network, mentors can serve as trusted guides. Their support helps individuals traverse the often-complex mental health landscape by facilitating access to appropriate resources and services. Mental health professionals can provide specialized treatment and clinical expertise, while community organizations can offer practical assistance, advocacy, and educational outreach.

Communities can build a comprehensive, holistic approach to addressing mental health needs. By fostering collaboration, mentors help leverage the unique strengths of each stakeholder, particularly in the context of grief. This supportive network can engender a sense of belonging, reduce stigma, and empower individuals to prioritize their mental well-being, ultimately fostering more resilient, thriving communities.

In the face of a growing global mental health pandemic, exacerbated by the unprecedented challenges and losses brought about by events like the COVID-19 pandemic, the role of mentors in bridging the gap to mental health support has become increasingly vital. Mentors' roles extend far beyond simply offering emotional support. They guide mentees to professional help, if needed. They direct them through the often-overwhelming mental health system. They encourage them through the help-seeking process. Collaboration between mentors and mental health professionals is essential for fostering a continuum of care with a coordinated approach to supporting mentees' mental health journeys.

To maximize their effectiveness, it is crucial to invest in building mentor competency through comprehensive training and education. We must leverage mentors as valuable resources. We must encourage their advocacy for mental health awareness and destigmatization efforts. Ultimately, the powerful network of support for grief and all mental health issues hinges on integrating mentorship into broader community.

PART III

GRIEF IN DIFFERENT CONTEXTS

CHAPTER 8

GRIEF AND YOUTH

THE SILENT PANDEMIC OF MENTAL health is a pervasive issue that affects individuals from all walks of life. However, one demographic particularly vulnerable to the challenges of mental health and the devastating impact of grief is our youth.

YOUTH MENTAL HEALTH

Young people today face a myriad of pressures and stressors. Beyond family dynamics and academic expectations, they now face more complex societal pressures because of social media. These factors can take a significant toll on their mental well-being. The result has been increased rates of anxiety, depression, and other mental health concerns.

When we add to this the profound grief that comes with losing a loved one, the impact on youth mental health can be even more severe. The loss of a parent, sibling, friend, or other close relationship can shatter a young person's sense of security and stability, leaving them grappling with intense emotions and existential questions.

For many young people, the COVID-19 pandemic only exacerbated these challenges. Its impacts are still evident in our communities. Not only did youth face the same fears and uncertainties as adults during this global crisis, but they also had to navigate disruptions to their education, social connections, and support systems. Many also experienced the heartbreaking loss of loved ones due to the virus, compounding their grief and mental health struggles.

In the face of these challenges, it is more important than ever that we prioritize the mental health of our youth. We must provide them with the support they need to cope with grief and build resilience. A powerful tool in this effort is mentoring.

For grieving people of any age, mentoring relationships can provide invaluable guidance, emotional support, and a sense of connection. For young people who may not have the same life experience or coping skills as adults, the presence of a caring mentor can be especially crucial.

Today's youth face unique mental health challenges, particularly in the context of grief and loss. For young people struggling with these issues, mentoring can extend a lifeline. Beyond providing them with support and guidance, mentors can invite the hope they need to weather the storm and emerge stronger on the other side.

Youth mental health includes their emotional, psychological, and social well-being. It encompasses the young person's ability to cope with stress, form relationships, and navigate the challenges of life. Unfortunately, many young people experience mental health problems such as anxiety, depression, self-esteem issues, and suicidal ideation.

Many factors contribute to youth mental health issues. Academic pressures, social media influence, family dynamics, trauma, and societal expectations may impact them differently than they would adults. In many cases, such pressures can mar their overall quality of life.

SUPPORT FOR YOUTH

Although we have looked at the benefits of mentoring in the previous section of this book, a particular focus on the benefits that mentoring has on youth mental health is important here. The benefits include:

DIRECT EMOTIONAL SUPPORT

Emotional support is a crucial aspect of mentoring that can greatly benefit young individuals facing mental health challenges. Mentoring relationships provide a safe and non-judgmental space for mentees to express their thoughts, feelings, and concerns.

Emotional support from a mentor reduces feelings of isolation. While such isolation can occur with adults and youth alike, it is especially prevalent among youth, especially those with few life experiences to deal with these challenges. Mentors who actively listen and empathize help reassure mentees that they are not alone in their struggles. Mentors can also provide validation by acknowledging the mentee's emotions and experiences, helping them feel understood and accepted.

Furthermore, mentors can guide mentees in navigating their emotions and coping with mental health challenges. They can share their own experiences, providing reassurance that overcoming such challenges is possible. Mentors can offer practical strategies for managing stress, anxiety, and depression, which helps mentees develop healthier coping mechanisms. They may introduce relaxation techniques, encourage self-care practices, or suggest professional resources that can further support the mentee's emotional well-being.

The emotional support provided by mentors might also contribute to the prevention and early intervention of mental health issues. By creating an open and supportive environment, mentors may be more likely to identify signs of distress or changes in a mentee's behavior. This early detection can prompt timely intervention, such as seeking professional help or connecting the mentee with appropriate mental health resources. By fostering open conversations and promoting help-seeking behaviors, mentors play a vital role in reducing the stigma associated with mental health.

EXTENDED SUPPORT

Especially with youth, it is essential for mentors to establish boundaries and recognize their limitations in providing emotional support. I have had first-hand experience where a youth I was mentoring overstepped the boundaries and had to be reminded what was acceptable and what was not. I have also been in situations where I knew my mentees' needs were beyond my limitations, and I had to recommend them to other services.

Mentors should be knowledgeable about available mental health resources and be prepared to refer mentees to professionals when necessary—especially when their mentees' needs exceed the level of support they can offer. Collaborating with mental health professionals and involving them in the mentoring program can ensure a comprehensive approach to supporting mentees' emotional well-being.

BENEFITS FOR YOUTH

Mentoring youth can often prove more immediately beneficial to youth than to adults. Beyond the emotional support they draw from the mentoring adult, they learn coping skills and develop healthy habits that can help them for a lifetime.

RESILIENCE BUILDING

Building resilience is a fundamental aspect of mentoring programs that significantly benefits young individuals facing adversity and mental health challenges. Resilience refers to the ability to adapt, recover, and bounce back from difficult experiences, setbacks, and stressors. Mentoring relationships provide a supportive environment where mentors can help young mentees develop resilience by sharing personal experiences, coping strategies, and problem-solving techniques.

A primary way mentors contribute to building resilience is through sharing their own experiences. Mentors can openly discuss their past challenges, and setbacks, and how they managed to overcome them. This shows youth that they too can navigate and overcome obstacles. These narratives provide hope and reassurance, demonstrating that setbacks and adversity are part of life's journey and can be overcome with determination and perseverance.

The mentor needs to know when it is timely to story share their life experiences and what stories they will share. The technique requires having the ability to relay a story that is relevant to the situation at hand. Sharing a story or experience that is not relevant is pointless as it only adds to the anxiety that the youth may be experiencing.

In addition to personal experiences, mentors can also introduce mentees to a range of coping strategies and techniques. They can teach mentees various tools for managing stress, anxiety, and other mental health challenges. These strategies may include relaxation techniques like deep breathing or engaging in physical activities that promote well-being. Mentors can also encourage mentees to develop healthy habits such as maintaining a balanced lifestyle, practicing self-care, and seeking social support when needed. This will empower them to proactively manage their stress and navigate challenges effectively.

Furthermore, mentors play a crucial role in developing problem-solving skills in mentees. By encouraging mentees to approach problems with a positive mindset, they help youth develop critical thinking and creativity. Mentors can guide mentees through the process of identifying problems, analyzing potential solutions, and making informed decisions. By teaching mentees problem-solving techniques, mentors enhance their mentees' ability to overcome challenges, build confidence, and develop a sense of self-efficacy.

Mentoring relationships also provides a valuable source of support and encouragement during challenging times. Mentors serve as trusted confidants, providing a listening ear and guidance when mentees encounter obstacles. They can help mentees reframe setbacks as opportunities for growth and learning, encouraging them to view challenges from a more positive perspective. This support helps mentees build trust— in themselves and others—by fostering a belief in their abilities to overcome adversity and reinforcing their sense of self-worth. These skills, in turn, can rebuild their confidence on others and the world that might have been shattered by their grief.

It is important to note that building resilience is a gradual process that takes time and practice. Mentoring programs should provide ongoing support and reinforcement, allowing mentees to develop and strengthen their resilience over time. Regular meetings, check-ins, and goal-setting can help mentors and mentees track progress and adjust strategies as needed.

Ultimately, by fostering resilience, mentoring programs equip young individuals with valuable skills and attitudes that extend beyond their immediate challenges. The resilience developed through mentoring can positively impact various aspects of mentees' lives, including their mental health, academic performance, relationships, and future success. It instils in them a belief in their ability to overcome adversity and face life's challenges with confidence, adaptability, and determination.

Increased Self-Esteem

Building and nurturing self-esteem is a crucial aspect of mentoring programs, and mentors have a significant impact on the self-esteem and self-confidence of mentees. Self-esteem refers to the overall subjective evaluation of one's worth and capabilities, while self-confidence relates to the belief in one's own abilities to succeed and accomplish goals. Mentoring relationships provide a supportive and empowering environment for mentees to develop a positive self-image and belief in their abilities.

Mentors play a vital role in boosting self-esteem by providing positive reinforcement and recognition of mentees' strengths and accomplishments. Mentors acknowledge and celebrate the achievements, efforts, and progress made by mentees, no matter how small. This helps them to foster a sense of pride and confidence in their abilities.

Furthermore, mentors actively work to build self-esteem by helping mentees identify and develop their unique talents. Mentors provide support as mentees explore different interests, hobbies, and skills. They encourage mentees to pursue activities that align with their strengths, which helps mentees gain a sense of competence and accomplishment. Developing a belief in their ability to succeed in specific areas builds in mentees a positive self-image.

Mentors also play a crucial role in encouraging personal growth and development in mentees. They provide guidance to help mentees achieve both short-term and long-term goals. In this process, mentors help mentees identify their aspirations so they can work towards them. Along the way, mentees grow in motivation and learn personal accountability for their success. As mentees make progress towards their goals, their self-confidence naturally grows, as they realize their ability to accomplish what they set out to do.

In addition to providing positive reinforcement and encouraging personal growth, mentors also serve as role models for positive self-esteem. Mentors demonstrate healthy self-esteem through their own actions, behaviors, and attitudes. As mentors assert themselves with self-assurance and self-respect, they inspire mentees to emulate these qualities. Mentors also promote a growth mindset, emphasizing the importance of learning from failures. Helping mentees interpret setbacks as opportunities for growth alters mentees' perspectives so individual events no longer define their worth.

Mentoring relationships offer a safe space for mentees to explore their thoughts and feelings without fear of judgment. Mentors actively listen to mentees, provide empathetic support, and validate their experiences. Such validation builds mentees' self-esteem by fostering a sense of belonging and acceptance. Mentors help mentees recognize their inherent worth by teaching them to value themselves, regardless of external validation or societal expectations.

Self-esteem building is an ongoing process that requires consistent support and reinforcement, which is especially important when dealing with grief. Mentors should provide continuous encouragement, regular check-ins, and opportunities for mentees to reflect on their progress. Mentors can also encourage mentees to engage in self-reflection and practice positive self-talk. Helping them challenge negative self-perceptions leads to their developing a more positive self-image.

ACADEMIC SUCCESS

Academic support encourages academic success. Such support is a key component of many mentoring programs. It often has a profound impact on the mental health and well-being of young individuals.

Academic support could be most needed when dealing with grief. Mentoring relationships that incorporate academic assistance provide valuable resources and strategies to help mentees improve their academic performance, increase engagement, and reduce the stress associated with educational challenges.

One of the most useful types of academic support is helping mentees develop effective study skills. These go hand-in-hand with useful time management techniques. Mentors can guide mentees in organizing study materials, creating study schedules, and implementing effective study strategies. Mentors can also assist mentees in setting realistic academic goals and developing action plans to achieve them. They can work with mentees to leverage their strengths as well as identify areas needing improvement. Mentors can follow such insights with strategies to leverage strengths and address weaknesses.

Mentors can further support mentees in identifying and accessing additional academic resources. This may include recommending resources, online tutorials, or educational websites. Going one step further, mentors can also connect mentees with academic support services available within their educational institutions.

In addition to academic skills, mentors can also assist mentees in developing effective problem-solving and critical-thinking skills. These skills are essential for overcoming academic challenges and navigating complex tasks. Mentors can help mentees analyze problems, explore different perspectives, and develop creative solutions.

Improved academic performance and engagement can positively impact mentees' mental health outcomes. Academic challenges and perceived academic failure can contribute to stress, anxiety, and low self-esteem in young individuals, which can be compounded with grieving the loss of a loved one or friend.

SOCIAL CONNECTION

Social connection is a vital aspect of mentoring relationships that significantly contributes to the overall well-being of young individuals. Mentoring programs offer mentees an opportunity to develop meaningful connections and expand their social networks. Once developed, these networks can help mentees foster a sense of belonging. Finding support can also enhance their overall life satisfaction.

Mentoring relationships provide a unique platform for mentees to establish a positive connection with their mentors. Mentors serve as role models, confidants, and sources of guidance, offering a trusted relationship where mentees can freely express themselves. Through regular meetings where they discuss shared experiences, mentors and mentees develop a bond based on trust, respect, and mutual understanding. This connection provides mentees with a reliable source of emotional support. The security encouraged by such support is essential for mental well-being.

Mentoring programs often involve group activities that bring together mentees participating in the program. These interactions invite mentees to connect with their peers, potentially fostering a sense of camaraderie. Building positive relationships with fellow mentees creates a supportive community where mentees can relate to one another, share challenges, and celebrate achievements. This social connection helps combat feelings of isolation and loneliness, two significant risk factors for poor mental health.

The sense of belonging that emerges from mentoring relationships and connecting with peers is crucial for mental health. Humans are social beings. A lack of social connection can lead to feelings of alienation, low self-esteem, and increased vulnerability to mental health issues. By providing mentees with a supportive network of mentors and peers, mentoring programs offer a sense of belonging, acceptance, and inclusion, which are essential protective factors for mental well-being.

In addition, the social connections developed through mentoring programs can extend beyond the program itself.

Mentees may establish long-lasting relationships with their mentors, continuing to seek support even after the formal mentoring period ends. Mentors can provide mentees with valuable social capital, introducing them to new networks, opportunities, and resources that can contribute to their overall life satisfaction.

Furthermore, the social connections formed through mentoring relationships can have positive effects on various areas of mentees' lives, including their academic performance and career development. Mentees who feel socially connected and supported are more likely to engage actively in their educational pursuits, seek out opportunities for growth, and develop a sense of direction that gives their life purpose.

Mentoring programs that foster supportive and inclusive environments maximize the benefits of social connection. Such programs should promote open communication, respect, and empathy among mentors and mentees. Group activities, workshops, or mentor-mentee pairings based on shared interests or backgrounds can further enhance the sense of connection and belonging. Additionally, creating opportunities for mentees to engage with mentors and peers outside of formal mentoring sessions, such as social events or group projects, can strengthen the social bonds and facilitate the development of lasting connections.

FINDINGS ON YOUTH MENTORSHIP

In 2016, the National Mentoring Resource Center published an analytical review that scrutinized the body of research pertinent to mentoring programs designed for young individuals grappling with mental health issues.

The review delved into 25 research studies, seeking to unravel the key questions associated with mentoring interventions for young individuals facing mental health challenges. Though the pool of research is somewhat limited and exhibits varied results, the review elucidates several intriguing findings:

- Mentoring programs have a positive impact on Youth with Mental Health Challenges (YMHC), especially those that are well-structured. The effect is particularly pronounced for higher-functioning children, such as those receiving outpatient mental health services or those identified with mental health-related challenges yet managing to remain in standard educational settings. Programs specifically targeting children and teenagers with Attention Deficit Hyperactivity Disorder (ADHD) also fare well.

- Substantial evidence suggests that participation in mentoring programs yields stronger positive effects on mental health and academic performance among YMHC.

- The efficacy of mentoring is influenced by certain individual and program-specific factors. For instance, youngsters displaying more severe symptoms appear to benefit more from mentoring. Moreover, structured, formal mentoring programs tend to be more effective than informal, naturally occurring mentorship.

- Among the transformative pathways through which mentoring aids YMHC are the reduction in caregivers' stress levels and the enhancement of the mentees' capacity to build trust and regulate emotions.

RECOMMENDATIONS FOR YOUTH MENTORSHIP

In light of these findings, the review furnishes practitioners with a set of recommendations aimed at optimizing their interventions by taking into account the available research. Practitioners are encouraged to:

- Develop a deeper understanding of how traumas and adverse life experiences have impacted the youth in order to tailor the services to meet their specific needs.

- Facilitate deeper engagement between the youth and their families and the required mental health services.

- Focus on designing program activities and mentor training that underscore the significance of fostering relationships and the mediating factors that drive outcomes.

- Establish clear criteria that define what constitutes success in the context of serving youth with mental health challenges and implement measurement strategies accordingly.

Beyond these highlights, this review offers a wealth of research-based information and actionable ideas for those looking to begin to serve YMHC more intentionally in their programs or, if they are already doing so, to strengthen existing practices. By looking at the research provided from this study, we can apply it from a practice perspective, a direction we should ideally go.

Understanding grief and how it impacts our youth is an important step moving forward. Even at an early age, they need the right coping mechanisms to navigate different life experiences they may encounter.

Ensuring that we have a solid process in place for mentoring youth who are struggling with mental health is very important. Knowing when it is time to listen and hear versus speak is one thing we need in place. I have found that many people are more inclined to speak than listen. We must reverse this inclanation for their mental health journey. Youth are more receptive when they feel they are being heard rather than being told what to do to fix their problem. Because they also need to be heard, we mentors must listen to their issues, which may include the loss of a loved one. Together, mentors and mentees must work together to resolve them.

Ultimately, I hope we can collectively work towards creating a world where no young person has to suffer in silence, where the pain of grief is met with compassion and understanding, and where every youth has access to the support they need to thrive in the face of life's challenges.

CHAPTER 9

GRIEF IN THE WORKPLACE

B EFORE I DELVE INTO THE main content of this chapter, I want to share a personal experience of dealing with grief in the workplace. It's a memory that has been etched indelibly into the depths of my psyche—the horrific moment when a promising young man, a close friend of mine, tragically ended his own life. His parents, consuming alcohol to great lengths, overlooked their son's extraordinary achievement of being chosen for the community adult hockey team. It was a moment of success that should have been celebrated, recognized, and appreciated. Instead, it was met with indifference and the hollow echo of their inebriation.

When he came home, brimming with excitement and anticipation of the praise he longed for, he found no one waiting to share his joy, no one to bask in his triumphant moment. His joy wilted in the cold silence of his parents' oblivion, leaving him with a sharp sense of loneliness and despair.

What followed was a gut-wrenching grief I could barely comprehend. He took his own life. To make matters even more unbearable, as one of two police officers in this small community, I was required to investigate his suicide. The stark reality of my friend's tragic end and the obligation to delve deeper into his death was a double blow, causing an irreparable tear in the fabric of my emotional well-being. I felt the world's weight on my shoulders, a crushing pressure that was almost unbearable.

As part of the investigation, I was required to transport his body to the closest morgue, in the back of the police vehicle, some eight hours away by gravel road in minus 40-degree weather. I was fortunate to have Debra, who was then my soon-to-be wife, travel with me. My boss didn't want me to go alone and was reluctant to leave the community. Debra drew the short straw and was volunteered to go with me on the long trip. On a positive note, this gave Debra the chance to see inside the life of a police officer's wife and what we had to deal with together. Debra was able to deal with the experience with minimal trauma and was a person I could talk with and share what I was feeling as we travelled to and from our home community. I tried to shield her from the majority of the trauma as I didn't want to scare her away. As I said to my parents many times, she was "a keeper" and I intended to have a long life with her.

On a grander scale, I found the geographical isolation only compounded my despair. Sometimes, I shifted my despair to Debra. Dealing with my behavior changes forced us to come together so we could attempt to handle the trauma together. Under most circumstances before Debra, I had no one to confide in. I couldn't share the trauma I was experiencing or debrief after each experience. Further, there were no professional services to deal with grief at work. In these moments of desperate loneliness, I found false solace in the biting burn of scotch whiskey, using it to buffer the unimaginable trauma that had engulfed my life. I was convinced that the scotch was a better solution than death by suicide. Debra deserved more than that.

The grief that consumed me at the loss of my young friend was not an isolated event but a distressingly common occurrence I faced repeatedly throughout my tenure in law enforcement. Ill-prepared for the emotional onslaught that our profession demanded, we were left to grapple with our demons with little to no support. The existing structures were inadequate, forcing us to seek refuge in destructive habits. For some, it was the numbing allure of alcohol; for others, the false escape of drugs; and tragically, for a few, the seemingly only way out was through the irreversible decision of suicide.

To this day, there are invisible yet deeply insidious triggers that have the power to launch me back into the churning ocean of grief. Like seismic waves, they strike without warning, stirring the deep-seated emotions beneath the surface. Each wave drags me back into the depths of that painful past, forcing me to relive the feelings of loss and despair all over again. It is a constant reminder of the unspeakable grief that my friend's suicide evoked, a memory that still haunts me.

So, why is exploring grief in the workplace relevant in this book? Because grief is not reserved for our personal lives. When an employee faces the loss of a loved one, the emotional and practical challenges can profoundly impact their well-being, focus, and productivity. Navigating the complexities of grief while simultaneously managing professional responsibilities can be an overwhelming and isolating experience.

For organizations, addressing the impact of grief on their workforce is not just a matter of compassion; it is a strategic imperative that can have far-reaching consequences on employee retention, morale, and overall company culture. Organizations can foster a culture of empathy, resilience, and loyalty by providing comprehensive support and resources to employees who are grieving, ultimately positioning themselves as employers of choice in an increasingly competitive job market.

This chapter, therefore, explores the vital importance of organizational support for employees who are facing loss, delving into the business case for implementing grief-sensitive policies and practices, as well as practical strategies for creating a compassionate and supportive work environment that prioritizes the well-being of its employees.

UNDERSTANDING GRIEF IN THE WORKPLACE

To effectively support employees who are grieving, it is crucial for organizations to develop a deep understanding of the unique challenges and experiences that grief can present in the workplace.

Grief is a complex and multifaceted experience that can manifest in various ways, both emotionally and practically.

Emotionally, grieving employees may experience a range of intense emotions, including sadness, anger, guilt, and anxiety. These emotions can fluctuate unpredictably, leading to periods of heightened distress or difficulty concentrating. Additionally, the experience of grief can be compounded by external factors, such as the nature of the loss, the relationship with the deceased, and the individual's personal coping mechanisms.

Practically, employees may face a multitude of logistical challenges, such as arranging funeral services, managing legal and financial affairs, and navigating complex family dynamics. These practical demands can create additional stress and strain, further impacting an employee's ability to maintain their usual level of productivity and focus.

It is important for organizations to recognize that the impact of grief is not limited to the individual employee. Grief can have a ripple effect across teams and departments, affecting morale, communication, and overall workplace dynamics. Colleagues may struggle to provide appropriate support or may inadvertently say or do things that are insensitive or hurtful to the grieving employee.

Moreover, organizations must acknowledge the diversity of grief experiences within their workforce. Cultural, religious, and personal beliefs can shape how individuals perceive and navigate grief. Employees need inclusive, respectful support mechanisms that accommodate a range of perspectives and traditions.

Organizations can better equip themselves to provide comprehensive and tailored support to their employees by developing a deeper understanding of the multifaceted nature of grief and its potential impact on the workplace, thereby fostering a culture of empathy, resilience, and mutual respect.

DEVELOPING A COMPREHENSIVE BEREAVEMENT POLICY

A foundational component of organizational support for grieving employees is the establishment of a comprehensive and compassionate bereavement policy. This policy should outline clear guidelines and provisions for employees who are facing the loss of a loved one. It must ensure they receive the necessary time, resources, and accommodations to navigate their grief journey while maintaining their professional responsibilities.

An effective bereavement policy should include flexible, inclusive leave provisions that account for the diverse range of relationships and situations that employees may encounter. Traditional policies that narrowly define eligible relationships or impose rigid time constraints can be insensitive and fail to address the complexities of grief.

Instead, organizations should strive to create policies that are adaptable and responsive to individual circumstances. This may involve offering a combination of paid and unpaid leave options, as well as the opportunity for employees to take intermittent or reduced schedules to accommodate their evolving needs.

Additionally, bereavement policies should consider the varying types of loss employees may experience, such as the death of a spouse, child, parent, or other close family member or friend. Different types of loss may require different levels of support and accommodation. Policies should be designed to address these nuances.

Beyond leave provisions, comprehensive bereavement policies should also outline additional resources and support services available to grieving employees. This may include access to counseling services, grief support groups, flexible work arrangements, and educational materials on coping strategies and self-care practices.

Organizations can demonstrate their commitment to supporting employees through difficult times by developing a comprehensive and compassionate bereavement policy. Such policies not only provide practical assistance but also send a powerful message that the organization prioritizes the well-being of its employees. Fostering such a culture of empathy ultimately contributes to increased loyalty, retention, and overall workplace satisfaction.

CREATING A SUPPORTIVE WORKPLACE CULTURE

While a robust bereavement policy is a crucial foundation, creating a truly supportive workplace culture for grieving employees requires a multifaceted approach that encompasses open communication, grief sensitivity training, and the promotion of mental health awareness.

Open communication is essential for creating an environment where employees feel comfortable sharing their experiences and seeking support when needed. This can be facilitated through regular check-ins, team meetings, and dedicated channels for employees to express their needs and concerns. Organization leaders at all levels should model vulnerability and authenticity, encouraging open dialogue about grief and its impact on both personal and professional lives.

Grief sensitivity training for management can equip them with skills to respond appropriately and sensitively to the needs of grieving employees. This training should cover topics such as active listening, empathetic communication, and understanding diverse cultural and personal perspectives on grief.

Promoting mental health awareness and reducing stigma surrounding grief and loss is also crucial for creating a supportive workplace culture. Organizations can achieve this by integrating mental health education into their employee wellness programs, providing resources and information on coping strategies, and fostering a safe and non-judgmental environment where employees feel empowered to seek help without fear of repercussions.

By cultivating a workplace culture that values open communication, grief sensitivity, and mental health awareness , organizations can create an environment where employees feel supported, understood, and empowered to navigate their grief journey with dignity and compassion.

OFFERING EMPLOYEE ASSISTANCE PROGRAMS

In addition to a comprehensive bereavement policy and a supportive workplace culture, organizations should invest in robust employee assistance programs (EAPs) that include resources specifically tailored to the needs of grieving employees.

EAPs can provide access to professional counseling services, grief support groups, and educational resources on coping strategies and self-care practices. These resources can be invaluable for employees navigating the emotional complexities of grief. Offering professional guidance is a way to create a safe space for them to process their experiences.

Furthermore, organizations should consider offering flexible work arrangements to accommodate grieving employees. Options may include remote work, flexible scheduling, or temporary adjustments to workloads and responsibilities. By providing these accommodations, organizations can alleviate some of the practical challenges faced by grieving employees. This flexibility allows them to focus on their healing process while maintaining their professional obligations.

Educational resources or training on grief and coping strategies can also be invaluable for employees. Organizations can provide access to online resources, workshops, or support materials that offer insights into the grieving process. It can also offer more general tips for self-care or guidance on how to support colleagues who are grieving. Demonstrating an organization's commitment to the well-being of their employees creates a supportive environment that promotes healing, resilience, and a sense of community during difficult times.

SUPPORTING GRIEVING EMPLOYEES THROUGH TRANSITIONS

One of the most challenging aspects of navigating grief in the workplace is the transition period when an employee returns to work after a period of bereavement leave. This transition can be fraught with emotional and practical challenges, requiring thoughtful, compassionate support from the organization.

Upon returning to work, grieving employees may experience a range of emotions, from anxiety and uncertainty to a sense of detachment or overwhelming sadness. It is crucial for organizations to provide a supportive, environment during this transition period by offering accommodations as needed.

Accommodations may involve temporarily adjusting workloads, responsibilities, or schedules to allow the employee to gradually re-acclimate to their professional responsibilities. Facilitating open communication with colleagues and clients can also help manage expectations to ensure a smooth transition back into the workplace.

Management plays a pivotal role in supporting grieving employees during this transition period. Company leaders should receive training on how to have sensitive and compassionate conversations, set realistic goals and expectations, and provide ongoing support and check-ins as needed.

Additionally, organizations should consider offering resources and support for colleagues of grieving employees. This may include guidance on how to sensitively welcome their co-worker back, how to provide appropriate support and boundaries, and how to navigate any potential changes or adjustments in team dynamics or workloads.

CARING FOR CAREGIVERS

While much of the focus on grief in the workplace centers around the loss of a loved one, it is equally important for organizations to support employees who are caring for terminally ill family members or friends. These caregivers often face immense emotional as well as practical challenges that can profoundly impact their well-being and their ability to perform their professional duties.

Caring for a terminally ill loved one can be an emotionally draining, physically taxing experience. Employees may feel anxious, sad, even overwhelmed as they navigate the complexities of managing care, making difficult decisions, and preparing for the eventual loss of their loved one.

Organizations should provide comprehensive support and resources for these caregiving employees. Flexible work arrangements, access to counseling services, and practical assistance with tasks such as coordinating care or managing medical appointments could prove invaluable to the employee and, in turn, to the company.

Additionally, it is crucial to address the risk of compassion fatigue and burnout among caregiving employees. Organizations can offer respite programs, support groups, and educational resources on self-care strategies to help caregivers maintain their emotional and physical well-being during this demanding time. This support can have a profound impact on employee loyalty, retention, and overall job satisfaction.

BUILDING A RESILIENT AND COMPASSIONATE WORKFORCE

Beyond supporting individual employees who are grieving or caring for loved ones, organizations have an opportunity to cultivate a broader culture of compassion within their workforce. By fostering an environment where grief and loss are openly discussed and understood, organizations can create a more supportive, inclusive workplace for all employees.

Promoting work-life balance through self-care builds a resilient workforce. Organizations can educate employees on everything from stress management techniques to mindfulness practices. Taking time for personal renewal and rejuvenation helps everyone.

Additionally, organizations should actively promote a culture of empathy through peer support. This can involve initiatives such as employee resource groups, mentorship programs, or workshops on emotional intelligence and compassionate communication. By creating opportunities for employees to support one another, organizations cultivate community. A sense of belonging can be invaluable during times of grief.

Organizations should celebrate the resilience of their employees by acknowledging the perseverance it takes to navigate difficult life experiences while maintaining professional responsibilities. Such recognition can take many forms, from informal acknowledgments to formal awards or recognition programs.

By investing in initiatives that foster resilience, empathy, and compassion within their workforce, organizations can create a supportive, inclusive environment that not only benefits employees who are grieving, but also contributes to overall employee well-being, engagement, and productivity.

IMPLEMENTING GRIEF-SENSITIVE PRACTICES ACRESS THE ORGANIZATION

Supporting employees who are facing loss and grief is not solely the responsibility of human resources or employee assistance programs.

It requires a coordinated effort across all organizational functions and departments to truly embed grief-sensitive practices into the fabric of the company culture.

Within the human resources department, this may involve adapting policies to align with the organization's bereavement policies and support initiatives. Organizations might revise leave protocols, update employee handbooks and resources, and provide manager trainings on how to effectively support grieving employees.

Integrating grief support into broader employee wellness initiatives is another crucial step. This could involve partnering with mental health professionals. Management could bring in grief counselors to offer workshops. Employees could create facilitated support groups. The company could invest in educational resources on topics related to grief, loss, and coping strategies.

Organizations could also collaborate with community partners to enhance their grief support offerings. This may involve forging partnerships with local hospice organizations, bereavement centers, or non-profit organizations that specialize in grief support services.

Organizations should create open lines of communication that include feedback mechanisms to gather perspectives from employees who have experienced grief or loss. This feedback can be invaluable in identifying areas for improvement. By filling gaps of support, companies can ensure their grief-sensitive practices meet the unique needs of its workforce.

By implementing grief-sensitive practices across all organizational functions and departments, companies can create a truly comprehensive, holistic approach to supporting employees who are facing loss. Healing occurs best in a culture of compassion, resilience, and mutual support.

EVALUATING ORGANIZATIONAL GRIEF SUPPORT

As organizations invest time and resources into developing comprehensive grief support initiatives, it is crucial to evaluate the effectiveness of these efforts. Collecting data, often in the form of employee feedback, positions organizations to gauge the impact of their support strategies, identify areas for improvement, and continuously adapt their approach to better meet the evolving needs of their workforce.

Employee feedback is an important metric to track. This can be gathered through surveys, focus groups, or one-on-one interviews with employees who have utilized the organization's grief support services. Collecting qualitative data on their experiences, challenges, and suggestions for improvement can provide invaluable insights into the effectiveness of the support provided.

Through employee surveys, organizations can assess the broader impact of their grief support initiatives on key performance indicators such as productivity, employee retention, and overall company culture. Analyzing before-and-after metrics on data such as absenteeism and turnover rates or turnover data can quantify the positive impact of an organization's efforts to make a stronger business case for continued investment in these initiatives.

Furthermore, organizations should continuously adapt their grief support strategies in response to changing workforce demographics, cultural shifts, and evolving best practices in the field of grief support. This may involve engaging external consultants, participating in industry forums, or collaborating with academic institutions to stay abreast of the latest research and trends.

Overall, supporting employees who are facing the loss of a loved one is not just a matter of compassion; it is a strategic imperative that can have far-reaching implications for an organization's success and sustainability. Prioritizing the well-being of their workforce requires implementing comprehensive grief support initiatives. By sustaining a culture of empathy, organizations secure loyalty that positions them as employers of choice in an increasingly competitive job market.

As we navigate the complexities of grief and loss in the modern workplace, it is imperative that organizations step up and embrace their role in supporting employees through these challenging times. By doing so, they not only demonstrate their commitment to the well-being of their workforce, but also cultivate a culture of compassion that can translate into long-term success and sustainability.

Grief in the workplace is a unique experience that requires specific support and resources. The impact of grief extends beyond the individual employee. It can affect team dynamics, productivity, and company culture. Creating a supportive work environment requires active engagement from everyone. Comprehensive bereavement leave policies and EAP services are essential for supporting grieving employees. Organizations must take a culturally sensitive, inclusive approach to grief support that respects diverse experiences as well as employee needs.

Organizations must prioritize grief support as a critical component of their employee support strategies. By investing in comprehensive policies, resources, and training, organizations can create a work environment that helps employees navigate the challenges of loss. In so doing, it will build a more resilient and compassionate workplace culture.

CHAPTER 10

GRIEF AND TRAUMA

G RIEF AND TRAUMA ARE TWO of life's most challenging experiences, each capable of causing immense distress and disruption to an individual's well-being. While grief and trauma are distinct experiences, they often intersect, creating a complex web of emotional, psychological, and physical challenges. While the interchange between grief and trauma can compound one another, mental health professionals are continually developing strategies for healing.

UNDERSTANDING TRAUMA

Trauma is a deeply disturbing experience that overwhelms an individual's ability to cope. It can cause feelings of helplessness, diminish sense of self, and make it difficult to regulate emotions. Trauma can take many forms, including physical trauma (such as accidents or assaults), emotional trauma (such as abuse or neglect), and psychological trauma (such as witnessing a violent event or experiencing a natural disaster).

Trauma impacts mental health. Its effects on well-being can be extreme and long-lasting. Mental health challenges related to trauma include anxiety, depression, and post-traumatic stress disorder (PTSD).

It can also affect physical health. Often chronic pain, sleep disturbances, and weakened immune functions can be traced directly to a traumatic occurrence.

Acute trauma comes from a single, isolated event. Chronic trauma results from repeated or prolonged exposure to distressing experiences. Chronic trauma, in particular, can have a cumulative effect on well-being, leading to complex trauma responses that can be difficult to untangle.

THE INTERSECTION OF GRIEF AND TRAUMA

Grief and trauma often intersect in complex and mutually reinforcing ways. Grief, in itself, can be a form of trauma, particularly in cases of sudden or violent loss. The experience of losing a loved one can shatter your sense of safety. The result may be feelings of helplessness, fear, and despair.

At the same time, preexisting traumas can exacerbate the grieving process. For example, an individual who has experienced childhood abuse may later struggle to cope with the loss of a supportive friend or family member, as the loss triggers past traumas that reinforce feelings of abandonment or worthlessness.

The intersection of grief and trauma can create unique challenges for individuals seeking to heal. The compounded distress of these experiences can overwhelm an individual's coping mechanisms, leading to a sense of being "stuck" in the pain and unable to move forward.

TRAUMATIC LOSS

Traumatic loss refers to the experience of losing a loved one in sudden, violent, or otherwise traumatic circumstances. Examples of traumatic loss include homicide, suicide, accidents, and natural disasters. The nature of these losses can complicate the grieving process, as survivors must grapple not only with the pain of the loss itself, but also with the traumatic circumstances surrounding the death.

The psychological impact of traumatic loss on survivors can be severe and long-lasting. Survivors may experience intense feelings of guilt, anger, and despair, as well as intrusive thoughts or memories related to the traumatic event. They may also struggle with a shattered sense of safety. Feeling either vulnerable or hypervigilant, they may generalize their pain with an overall mistrust in the world.

Unique symptoms of trauma—from flashbacks to nightmares to avoidance behaviors—complicate the grieving process. These symptoms can interfere with our ability to engage in the tasks of grieving, such as accepting the reality of the loss and adjusting to life without the deceased.

COLLECTIVE TRAUMA AND GRIEF

Collective trauma refers to the psychological and emotional impact of a traumatic event on an entire community or society. Examples of collective traumas include natural disasters, mass shootings, terrorist attacks, and pandemics. These events can shatter a community's sense of safety and stability. The result is often widespread feelings of fear, helplessness, and despair.

Collective traumas can shape individual and communal grief experiences in powerful ways. On the positive side, the shared nature of the trauma can create solidarity among survivors, as they grapple with the pain and loss together. Conversely, the scale and scope of the trauma can overwhelm a community's resources and coping mechanisms, leading to a sense of collective grief and mourning.

The COVID-19 pandemic is a recent example of a collective trauma that has had a profound impact on grief experiences worldwide. The pandemic not only caused widespread loss of life, but it also disrupted traditional grieving rituals and support systems, leaving many individuals feeling isolated and unsupported in their grief.

HISTORICAL AND INTERGENERATIONAL TRAUMA

Historical trauma is cumulative emotional and psychological wounding experienced by a group or community over generations, often as a result of systemic oppression, violence, or discrimination. Examples of historical trauma include the experiences of indigenous communities, the legacy of slavery and segregation, and the impact of the Holocaust on Jewish communities.

Intergenerational trauma refers to the ways in which the effects of historical trauma can be passed down from one generation to the next, even among those who did not directly experience the original traumatic events. This transmission can occur through a variety of mechanisms, including epigenetic changes, family dynamics, and cultural narratives.

The impact of historical and intergenerational trauma on grief experiences can be profound and complex. For individuals and communities grappling with the legacy of historical trauma, the experience of loss can trigger deep-seated feelings of anger, despair, and injustice. The grieving process may be complicated by a sense of collective mourning for the losses and injustices of the past, as well as a need to honor and remember those who have been lost.

Culture and identity play a significant role in shaping trauma responses, particularly in the context of historical and intergenerational trauma. For example, indigenous communities may draw on traditional healing practices or spiritual beliefs to cope with grief and trauma, while also grappling with the ongoing impact of colonialism and cultural erasure.

POST-TRAUMATIC STRESS DISORDER (PTSD) AND GRIEF

Post-Traumatic Stress Disorder (PTSD) can develop in the aftermath of traumatic events such as natural disasters, violent assaults, or military combat. Besides feelings of fear, anger, and detachment commonly associated with grief, PTSD symptoms encompass flashbacks, nightmares, avoidance behaviors, and hyperarousal.

PTSD and grief share a complex, multifaceted relationship. For those of us who have experienced traumatic loss, the presence of PTSD symptoms can complicate and prolong the grieving process. The intrusive thoughts and memories associated with PTSD can make it difficult for us to move through the grieving process.

At the same time, grief can exacerbate PTSD symptoms, particularly if the loss triggers memories of past traumas or reinforces feelings of helplessness and despair. This can create a vicious cycle in which grief and trauma symptoms feed into one another, making it difficult for individuals to find a path towards healing.

Strategies exist for simultaneously coping with PTSD and grief. Often a combination of therapy, medication, and self-care practices can be effective. Trauma-focused therapies, such as cognitive-behavioral therapy (CBT) and eye movement desensitization and reprocessing (EMDR), have proven particularly effective in addressing PTSD symptoms. Even when trauma intensifies the process toward healing, grief counseling helps sufferers process their loss and find meaning in the aftermath of trauma.

RESILIENCE AND POST-TRAUMATIC GROWTH

The ability to bounce back and adapt in the face of adversity is known as resilience. Post-traumatic growth refers to the positive psychological changes that can occur as a result of struggling with highly challenging life circumstances. While grief and trauma can be incredibly difficult experiences, they can also serve as catalysts for positive personal transformation.

Thanks in part to social support, those who've suffered trauma may discover lessons along their healing journey. With resilience, they can build on those lessons until they find a new path towards personal growth. Ultimately, that resilience can even spark in them a new sense of purpose or meaning.

Post-traumatic growth can take many forms. The road to recovery may lead to increased self-awareness, deepened relationships, and even a greater appreciation for life. For some individuals, the experience of grief and trauma can serve as a wake-up call that prompts them to reassess their priorities so they can better align their goals with their values.

It is important to note that resilience and post-traumatic growth are not universal experiences. Also, not all individuals will experience these positive changes in the aftermath of grief and trauma. Further, resilience that can lead to such affirming growth does not negate the pain and difficulty of these experiences. Rather, they serve as testaments to the human capacity for healing.

THE ROLE OF SUPPORT SYSTEMS

Social support plays a critical role in coping with grief and trauma. Besides offering emotional support during difficult times, a network of caring individuals often gives the grieving a sense of belonging.

Various types of support is particularly helpful when coping with grief and trauma. Professional counseling can provide a safe and confidential space for you to process your experiences and develop coping strategies. Support groups may invite a sense of connection and validation from others who have experienced similar traumas.

Community-based resources, such as faith-based organizations, community centers, and advocacy groups, can also play an important role in supporting you or your family when coping with trauma-induced grief. Besides giving emotional support, these organizations can also provide practical assistance for completing daily tasks. In some cases, they even supply financial support.

Accessing support can be particularly challenging for marginalized communities. Added barriers include language differences, cultural stigma, and systemic inequities. Efforts to support these communities must be culturally responsive. Grounding assistance in an understanding of the unique challenges and strengths of each community is paramount.

HEALING AND RECOVERY

The path towards healing and recovery from trauma-triggered grief is a deeply personal process. No one-size-fits-all approach helps everyone. What works for one person may not work for another. However, some common elements can support the healing process.

As described earlier, self-care refers to the practice of taking care of one's physical, emotional, and spiritual needs in the aftermath of a difficult experience. Basic practices include getting enough sleep, eating well, and exercising. More specific routines might entail meditating, journaling, or engaging in other forms of creative expression.

Self-compassion entails treating yourself with kindness, understanding, and, when necessary, forgiveness as you explore difficult emotions and face challenging experiences. Suffering is a part of the human experience. In even our darkest moments, we all deserve care and support, even from ourselves.

Meaning-making is the process of finding purpose in the aftermath of a traumatic experience. Often it requires grappling with difficult questions about the nature of life and death. In the process we may also find ways to honor those who we've lost. For some, meaning-making may involve activism or advocacy work. For others, it may spark a deep, introspective journey that deepens our spiritual or philosophical beliefs.

To heal from trauma, we must grapple with difficult emotions and face challenging experiences. Throughout the process, a commitment to self-compassionate self-care can have profound benefits. As important can be the support we seek from others. Those supporters can be individual counselors or support groups. Always, they also include caring relationships with family and friends.

The intersection of grief and trauma is complex. Compassion can help this sensitive, challenging journey. We get through it in part by a willingness to sit with difficult emotions or engage in experiences we might find uncomfortable. We can begin to develop strategies for healing that are grounded in both research and lived experience by understanding the ways these experiences can compound and complicate one another.

To work through grief from trauma, we all must prioritize the needs of those who are most impacted by these challenges. Individuals and entire communities who have experienced marginalization, oppression, and systemic inequities face unique barriers to accessing support and resources. Our support for them is essential to us all.

PART IV

MOVING FORWARD

CHAPTER 11

HONORING YOUR UNIQUE GRIEF JOURNEY

JUST AS NO TWO RELATIONSHIPS or connections are identical, the ways in which we experience and process grief are shaped by a multitude of factors. Our cultural backgrounds, our beliefs and values, our personal histories, and the specific circumstances surrounding our loss make everyone's grief journey unique.

In a world that often seeks to impose a one-size-fits-all approach to grief, or to prescribe a set of universal stages or timelines that we must adhere to, it is essential that we honor the inherent individuality of this sacred journey. For each of us, the path through grief will look different, with its own unique contours, ebbs, and flows, shaped by our lived experiences and the depth of our love for the one we have lost.

This chapter is a space to reflect on and embrace the nuances of your own grief journey, to explore the ways in which your loss has reshaped your sense of identity, your priorities, and your perspective on the world around you. It is an invitation to challenge societal narratives and expectations so that you can give yourself permission to grieve in your own authentic way, at your own pace, without judgment or the pressure to "move on" or "get over" your loss.

THE EBB AND FLOW OF GRIEF

A profound yet oft-overlooked aspect of grief is its inherently cyclical nature. Contrary to the linear models that are often presented, grief is not a straightforward progression from one stage to the next, with a clear beginning and end. Rather, it is a journey that ebbs and flows.

When you are grieving, this ebb and flow can disorient and overwhelm. Waves of sadness, anger, or yearning may wash over us, only to be followed by moments of calm or even joy. It is not uncommon to find ourselves caught in a constant push and pull, feeling as though we are making progress one day, only to be knocked sideways by a powerful swell of grief the next. Triggers, such as visiting a place special to a loved one you lost years after your loss, can throw you into a fit of sadness.

Yet within this cycle, you can find profound wisdom and beauty. The sudden new spike of sadness reminds us that grief is not a linear process to be "completed" or "resolved." Rather, it is a sacred journey inextricably woven into the rhythms of life itself.

YOUR GRIEF, YOUR PATH

In the face of loss, we should permit ourselves to grieve in our own unique and authentic ways, free from the constraints of societal expectations or cultural norms. While there may be rituals, practices, or traditions that hold meaning for us, we must also be willing to challenge and then redefine these constructs when they no longer resonate with our individual experiences.

For some, this may mean embracing emotional expression and vulnerability in ways that defy traditional gender roles or cultural norms. For others, it may involve creating entirely new rituals or practices that feel deeply personal, even if they diverge from the paths that have been laid before us.

Ultimately, we must navigate the path of grief on our own terms, intuitively guided by our own inner wisdom. This may mean embracing solitary periods of introspection. It may involve seeking out communities of support and shared understanding. It could involve expressing our grief through creative outlets like writing, art, or music. It may manifest in acts of service or philanthropy that honor the memory of our loved one.

Regardless of the specific shape our grief journey takes, what matters most is that we allow ourselves the freedom to explore and express our emotions without judgment or the pressure to conform to external expectations. By honoring the unique contours of our grief, we open ourselves to the possibility of profound healing and transformation.

THE HEALING IS IN THE JOURNEY

While grief is often associated with profound pain and sorrow, it is also a journey that holds immense potential for growth, self-discovery, and a deeper understanding of what it means to be human. For within the depths of our loss, we are invited to redefine our identities, our priorities, and our values in ways that can profoundly shift our perspectives and our relationship to the world around us.

For some, this process of redefining may involve letting go of superficial pursuits or societal expectations that no longer resonate. In their place, you may cultivate deeper connections with loved ones, pursue long-held passions, or engage in acts of service or activism that align with your values. Others of us may reevaluate the ways we have defined ourselves and our sense of purpose. In turn, we may feel inspired to explore new paths or possibilities that previously felt out of reach.

Regardless of the specific form this redefinition takes, there is profound power in allowing ourselves to be transformed by the experience of loss. By embracing the lessons and insights that emerge from our grief, we open ourselves to the possibility of living our lives with greater intentionality, authenticity, and a deeper appreciation for the preciousness of each moment.

INTEGRATING LOSS

Most profoundly, grief can teach us the importance of integrating loss into the fabric of our lives, rather than seeking to "move on" or "get over" our grief. This process of integration is not about letting go of our loved ones or the memories we hold dear; it is about finding ways to carry their legacies and their love forward with us, weaving their stories and their impact into the fabric of our ongoing lives. As we create space for both the sadness and the joy, the grief and the growth, we can acknowledge that these seemingly contradictory experiences as essential parts of being human.

For some, this integration may involve creating new rituals or traditions that honor the memory of their loved one, such as setting a place for them at the table during family gatherings or finding ways to incorporate their passions or values into our own daily lives. For others, it may involve cultivating an ongoing sense of connection or communication with our loved one. Some people continue to talk to their loved ones as if they are there to keep their connection going.

THE IMPORTANCE OF SELF-COMPASSION

Throughout the journey of grief, self-compassion is an essential guidepost worth practicing. Grief is a profoundly challenging and often exhausting experience. It demands immense emotional and physical resilience. The journey can leave us feeling raw, vulnerable, and at times, overwhelmed by the sheer weight of our loss.

During such moments, it is essential to extend compassion and kindness to ourselves. One simple way is to recognize that grieving requires some of the most difficult and sacred work we will ever undertake. Self-compassion may manifest in a variety of ways. We can allow ourselves to rest when we need it, seek support and guidance from others, even simply acknowledge the profound courage it takes to face each day in the wake of loss.

Self-compassion may also demand challenging the societal narratives and expectations that often surround grief, particularly the notion that we must "move on" or "get over" our loss within a prescribed timeline. To expect ourselves to "move on" or to reach a point of complete resolution is to deny the profound impact that loss has on our lived experiences.

Instead, self-compassion invites us to embrace a radical acceptance of our grief. Ironically, we can find comfort in honoring the depth of our pain and giving ourselves permission to feel and express the full range of our emotions without judgment or shame. By acknowledging there is no "right" way to grieve, we are free to be individuals on our own path instead of struggling to fit into a rigid course shaped by a myriad of personal, cultural, and contextual factors.

BUILDING YOUR SUPPORT NETWORK

While the journey of grief is profoundly personal, it is also a path that we need not walk alone. One of the most powerful sources of support in the grieving process can be found in seeking professional counseling or grief mentoring. These spaces provide a safe, non-judgmental environment to explore the complexities of our grief, to share our stories and experiences, and to find validation and understanding from others who have walked similar paths.

In addition to professional support, we are well served by cultivating a network of understanding listeners within our personal circles (friends, family members, or community members). Find supporters willing to bear witness to our grief without judgment or the need to "fix" or "resolve" our pain. Individually or in groups, they can serve as anchors of support who offer a compassionate presence and a willingness to simply hold space for our grief in all its messy, unpredictable forms.

Building this support network is not always easy, particularly in a society that often struggles with acknowledging and validating the depths of grief and loss. It may require us to step outside of our comfort zones. When we're brave enough to be vulnerable, we can ask for the support we need, even when it feels difficult or uncomfortable to do so.

Cultivating such support network is immensely rewarding. It reminds us we are not alone on this journey. We come to appreciate that our pain and our love are part of the universal human experience.

We find others who are willing to hold space for us as we navigate the ever-shifting terrain of loss.

NOURISHING MIND, BODY, AND SPIRIT

Grief demands immense emotional and physical resources from us. Sometimes the process leaves us feeling drained, exhausted, and at times, disconnected from our own sense of well-being. That makes it essential to nourish our mind, body, and spirit as we navigate the terrain of loss.

Grief can take a profound toll on our bodies. The stress and emotional turmoil of loss can manifest in a myriad of ways, from disrupted sleep patterns and changes in appetite, to chronic pain, headaches, and a weakened immune system. Throughout this time, we can counterbalance these depleting impacts by tending to our physical needs. Conscious efforts to nourish our bodies can be simple, but the effects profound. Eat nutritious foods. Get adequate hydration. Regularly engage in gentle movement or exercise.

Practices such as mindfulness meditation, yoga, or simply taking a walk in nature can also be powerful tools for nourishing our minds and spirits during the grieving process. These practices can help us cultivate a sense of presence and grounding. Even in the midst of our pain and sorrow, they can provide a much-needed respite from the emotional turbulence of grief.

For many, the grieving process can also be a time of profound spiritual exploration. It often leads us to grapple with existential questions around the meaning of life and death. In response, we may seek to find a new sense of purpose and connection within our loss. Helpful venues for such exploring such questions may involve recommitting to past spiritual or religious practices that have been meaningful in our lives. More often, it prompts us to explore new avenues of spiritual growth and understanding.

Nourishing our mind, body, and spirit during the grieving process is not about "fixing" or "resolving" our grief. Instead, we honor the profound demands that grief places upon us by providing ourselves with the resources and support we need to navigate this sacred journey with grace, resilience, and self-compassion.

THE CONTINUED BOND

The grieving journey affords us an opportunity to explore and deepen our connection with our loved ones, even in the face of their physical absence. For while death may separate us physically from those we have lost, the bonds of love and memory we share with them can transcend the boundaries of this life.

This concept of the "continued bond" invites us to reimagine our relationships with our loved ones in new and profoundly meaningful ways. When we recognize that the love we share does not end with death, our relationship with our loved one continues to evolve and transform. As we integrate the memories of our loved ones into daily living, we discover how our loved ones continue to impact our lives.

For some of us, this continued bond may manifest in the form of rituals or practices that honor the memory of our loved one. Simple rituals include setting a place for them at the table during family gatherings, lighting a candle in their honor on significant dates, or visiting places that held special meaning for them. More complex forms of inclusion may involve finding ways to incorporate your loved one's passions, values, or wisdom into your daily life. Doing so is a way of carrying forward their legacy.

Regardless of the specific form it takes, cultivating this continued bond engenders powerful solace and healing in the grieving process. By ensuring that their stories and their love continue to ripple outward, we honor the impact they continue to have on our lives.

Although we hold our loved ones and their memories in our hearts, we must ensure that this continued bond is not about clinging to the past or denying the reality of our loss. Instead, we integrate the memory and impact of our loved ones into the present moment as we continue to evolve on our own journey.

THE GIFTS IN ALLOWING GRIEF

While grief is undoubtedly one of the most challenging and painful experiences we can endure, it is also a journey that can ultimately lead us to profound gifts of insight, growth, and transformation. In the depths of our loss, we are invited to open ourselves to the mysterious complexities of the human experience. When we do, our perspectives can shift profoundly as we gain new understanding of ourselves and the world around us.

One generous gift grief can offer is the opportunity to cultivate a deeper sense of presence and appreciation for the preciousness of life. In the wake of loss, we are often jolted out of the routines and distractions that can so easily consume our daily lives. In their place, we are confronted with the stark reality of our own mortality and the fragility of the human experience. This confrontation can be a powerful catalyst for living with greater intentionality, savoring the beauty and joy that exists in each moment, and cultivating a profound sense of gratitude for the gift of life itself.

Grief can also be a powerful catalyst for creative self-expression that enhances personal growth. As we process the profound emotions that accompany loss, we may find ourselves drawn to creative pursuits such as writing, painting, or playing music. Art is a rich way to explore our souls. It can give voice to our grief. Creative expression can be profoundly healing. As we create art, the art transforms us.

Ultimately, grief's richest gift is the opportunity to embrace the full spectrum of the human experience. Acknowledging the depths of our pain and sorrow opens us to the profound beauty that can emerge from even the darkest moments of our lives. This journey invites us to surrender to the mysteries of life and death. When we embrace the cyclical nature of loss and rebirth, we can find solace in the knowledge that we are all part of a shared existence of love, loss, and growth that stretches across time and space.

LIVING LIFE IN GRIEF'S ERRANT RHYTHMS

Patience and self-compassion help us heal through the grieving process. To truly honor our grief, we must surrender to its rhythms. We must allow ourselves to feel the full depth of our pain, without judgment. As we learn to hold space for the contradictions and complexities that grief brings, we can embrace the moments of joy and laughter that may arise even in the midst of our deepest sadness.

This is not to say that the journey of grief is easy or without its challenges. Indeed, there will be times when the weight of our loss feels almost unbearable. When the path ahead seems shrouded in darkness and uncertainty, we have several healthful options. We can lean on our support networks. We can extend compassion to ourselves. We can remind ourselves that grief is a universal human experience. We are one among countless souls who have taken similar journeys throughout the ages.

Ultimately, to live life in grief's errant rhythms is to embrace the profound mysteries and complexities of the human experience. It requires acknowledging that loss and love, pain and joy, are all part of the intricate tapestry that weaves our lives together. Healing occurs as we surrender to the understanding that there is no "moving on" from grief. It is a process of integration where we learn to carry the weight of our loss while simultaneously making space for new experiences, new growth, and new ways of being in the world.

This journey is not an easy one, but it is a profoundly sacred one. This path has the power to shape us, to deepen our compassion and our understanding of our own humanity.

In the end, the journey through grief is one of the most powerful catalysts for personal growth and self-discovery that we may ever encounter. The journey strips us bare to confront the fragility of our existence and the profundity of our love. In doing so, it invites us to rebuild ourselves from the ground up. It encourages us to question the assumptions and narratives that have shaped our lives. In empowers us to redefine our priorities, our values, and our relationship to the world around us.

For many people, this process of redefinition leads to a newfound sense of purpose. It spurs a commitment to living life with greater intentionality and authenticity. While it may mean letting go of old identities, it also emboldens us to embrace new ways of being. It stirs new passions. It inspires pursuits that feel more aligned with the wisdom and insights gained through the depths of loss for others.

Regardless of the specific form this transformation takes, grief is not merely a journey of sorrow and pain, but also one of beauty, resilience, and growth. It is a path that has the power to break us open to the deepest truths of our existence, to reveal the boundless depths of our capacity for love, courage, and connection.

GRIEF REVISITED – RENEE FESSER'S STORY

Before closing this chapter, I wanted to take the opportunity to share a story with you about accepting grief as a natural part of our lives as human beings. The story is told by Renee Fesser herself and reads as follows:

> *Today I reflect on life and living. I am witness to the world's glorious splendour that is proof enough of a God above. I take solace in this and feel uplifted as I write. My writing is a daily practice of grounding and nurturing. As I write, I feel the spirit of love and equanimity move through me.*
>
> *My grief story is a shift in perspective regarding grief, and this has made all the difference.*
>
> *Grief arrived early in my life after the loss of a marriage, mixed with trauma and complication. This complication was not just the loss of a person, place, or thing; it was much deeper. The "complication" would both propel me forward and keep me frozen for years to come. This would come in waves, pushing a frozen iceberg through time and space, which is life.*
>
> *The most painful grief wasn't from the trauma, though; it was in the process of healing. You see, since trauma had me frozen and stuck, I was unable to have another relationship. At the time of writing this, I am still in the healing process, and this brings waves of grief, which I have learned to ride.*
>
> *When you heal, you receive gifts of awareness, and new pain arrives as you grieve the life that could have been. This grief is like no other; it is bone-deep and heart-wrenching.*

All you can do is ride the waves while moving forward, navigating new terrain and embracing fear.

Nevertheless, grief has gifted me with many gifts over time.

These gifts are tools, skills, strengths, and resources. In the early days of healing, I did not welcome grief. In my hurry to get on with life and heal, I took to learning, working, and caring for others. On the outside, I looked and acted like a fully functional and thriving woman, yet, beneath the surface, the pain and sorrow that I had banished were buried deep.

Thankfully, life allows us plenty of opportunities to heal. Healing occurs on many levels, and often when we think we are raw, weak, and at our lowest, we are in the muck of it all, giving us an opportunity to feel again. We must embrace the dark to experience the light. This means that we must get in touch with our deepest pain and lean into it in order to live fully. This is my daily practice.

My healing journey has just begun. Grief has gifted me with hope, grace, empathy, compassion and a new understanding of human suffering and resilience. Healing and life are a journey that is bittersweet and one we do not need to travel alone.

Alas, grief and I are no strangers. We have become old friends. Grief sits with me, holds me, and introduces me to new friends like hope and peace. I now welcome grief, for I know that grief is a part of life and healing. We need to feel it all. Grief has many layers, and yes, it is still unfolding.

Renee Fesser, BSW, RSW

CHAPTER 12

FINDING MEANING AND PURPOSE

THE PAIN OF LOSING A loved one can be utterly devastating. Shattered, we may question the very foundations of our existence. And yet, within this darkness lies the potential for profound transformation—a catalyst for personal growth where we discover our life's deeper meaning and purpose.

While grief is often associated with anguish, despair, and loss, it can also serve as a powerful force that awakens us to the preciousness of life. That awakening can inspire us to live with greater authenticity, intention, and purpose. The journey through grief is a deeply personal one. Its impact on each individual is unique. However, many who have walked this path have emerged not only intact but transformed. With a renewed appreciation for life, they reframe their priorities from a deeper connection to their core values.

THE SEARCH FOR MEANING

In the depths of grief, we are often confronted with existential questions that shake the very foundations of our beliefs and assumptions about life. The loss of a loved one can leave us feeling adrift. Untethered, we often question our purpose. We wonder about the meaning behind our existence. Although this experience can be profoundly disorienting and unsettling, it also presents an opportunity for self-reflection that leads to personal growth.

Grappling with the pain of loss leads many of us to reprioritize our values as we determine what truly matters in life. Trivialities that once consumed our attention may fade into insignificance. In their place will be deeper questions about our life's purpose. The legacy we want to leave can come into sharp focus. This search for meaning is a powerful catalyst for personal transformation. It encourages us to live more intentionally as we align our actions with our core values.

For some, this process may involve exploring spiritual or religious beliefs. We may seek solace in traditional or non-traditional practices. Others may find meaning by connecting with loved ones. Special bonding often occurs as we share cherished memories about the loved one we've lost. Our deeply personal search for meaning will likely require us to find the courage to confront our fears, doubts, and vulnerabilities. The result is often an open heart more adept at savoring each moment of life.

PERSONAL GROWTH AND SELF-DISCOVERY

Grief has a way of stripping away the layers of our personas, revealing our true selves in all their rawness and vulnerability. In this state of profound openness, we may uncover aspects of ourselves that were previously hidden or overlooked. The process can lead to profound personal growth and self-discovery.

As we navigate the tumultuous waters of grief, we may tap into inner strengths and resilience we never knew existed. The challenges we face can push us to our limits, forcing us to confront our fears and limitations head-on. In doing so, we may discover a newfound sense of courage, determination, and self-assurance that empowers us to tackle life's obstacles with greater fortitude.

Moreover, the process of grieving can foster a deeper self-awareness and emotional intelligence. As we confront the complex emotions associated with loss, we may gain a greater understanding of ourselves.

We learn our triggers, hone our coping mechanisms, and discover our capacity for growth and healing. Interpersonally, this heightened self-awareness can then translate into more meaningful relationships as we develop better communication skills. Intrapersonally, we gain a deeper appreciation for the nuances of the human experience.

SHIFTS IN PERSPECTIVE

Grief has a way of reframing our perspectives. It forces us to confront the fragility and impermanence of life. This shift in perspective can be both humbling and profoundly transformative. The reward is often a newfound appreciation for the present moment. In each of those moments, we may cultivate a deeper gratitude for the blessings in our lives.

As we emerge from the depths of grief, we may find ourselves living with greater mindfulness and intentionality. Irrelevant worries make way for a heightened awareness of what truly matters. Based on our values, we decide what that is. Our relationships? Our passions? Our impact on the world around us? Perhaps a combination of them define who we have become.

A shift in perspective goes hand-in-hand with re-evaluated priorities. Once we're clearer about our values, we are more likely to align our actions with our highest aspirations. We may make conscious choices to simplify our lives. Frequently we will prioritize self-care or pursue paths that bring us richer fulfillment.

Most encouragingly, the experience of loss can cultivate a profound sense of gratitude. We acknowledge deeper gratitude for the time we had with our loved ones, for the lessons they imparted, and for the gift of life itself. This gratitude can serve as a powerful antidote to the negative emotions that often accompany grief. They help us find joy and beauty in even the most trying of circumstances.

POST-TRAUMATIC GROWTH

While the term "post-traumatic growth" may seem counterintuitive in the context of grief, research has shown that individuals can experience positive psychological changes in the aftermath of trauma. Grief, in particular, can be a channel for profound transformation.

Post-traumatic growth results in developing new perspectives, building new strengths, and finding opportunities for growth that may not have been possible without the experience of trauma or loss. This growth is evident from multifaceted perspectives. We may feel increased personal strength. We develop a deeper appreciation for life. Our relationships can improve. Most abstractly, we might even develop a heightened sense of spirituality or existential awareness.

For many of us who have experienced grief, this growth emerges from a place of profound vulnerability once we acknowledge life's fragility. Confronting our own mortality and accepting the impermanence of their loved ones, we can find the courage to live life to its fullest.

As we foster a deeper appreciation for the present moment, we nurture a newfound gratitude for the relationships and experiences that enrich our lives. This shift in perspective can lead to more mindful living. With a greater investment in personal growth, we develop deeper connections to our values and purpose.

REDEFINING IDENTITY AND PURPOSE

Grief can prompt us to reevaluate our identities. The result often brings us a new life purpose. Navigating the complexities of loss leads many of us to question the paths we have chosen. We frequently answer that question by setting new goals that change the trajectory of our life.

Self-reflection can be both unsettling and liberating. It encourages us to shed the layers of expectations and societal norms that may have constrained our authentic selves. In the wake of grief, we may discover new passions, talents, and aspirations that were previously obscured by the demands of daily life.

For some of us, this journey leads to a complete shift in lifestyle. Aligning our actions with their deepest desires could lead us to change careers. We might find purpose in advocacy, philanthropy, or community service related to causes that resonate with our most cherished beliefs.

Regardless of the path we choose, redefining our identity can starkly change our life's purpose. In the aftermath of grief, acting on our new values can be a powerful act of self-affirmation. By embracing the lessons gained through loss, we often emerge with a renewed sense of authenticity. Finding new purpose gives us a deeper connection to our true selves.

THE ROLE OF SUPPORT SYSTEMS

Throughout our profoundly personal journey through grief, support systems play an essential part in facilitating our transformation. Grief can be an isolating experience. A strong network of support provides the emotional, practical, and psychological resources necessary to navigate this challenging terrain.

Professional help from counseling or therapy can be invaluable in processing complex emotions. These sessions provide opportunities for us to develop coping strategies. The process also enables us to gain insights into personal growth that lead to healing. Support groups, both in-person and online, create community. Connecting with others, especially those facing similar challenges, provides a safe space where mutual support thrives.

Mentorship can be instrumental in helping us find meaning and purpose in the wake of loss. A mentor who has walked a similar path can offer wisdom, perspective, and practical strategies for personal growth. They act as an inspiring beacon of hope for our transformation.

CULTIVATING MEANING AND LEGACY

Along the transformative journey of grief, we might find solace and purpose by creating a lasting legacy that honors the memory of our loved one. This can take various forms, from acts of service and philanthropy to creative pursuits and personal projects.

Some of us actively support causes that were meaningful to our loved ones. As we reclaim our sense of self independent of the loved one we lost, we may find fulfillment in creative outlets, such as writing, art, or music. Art invites us to express our grief while preserving the memory of our loved one.

Sharing our stories with others can be a fulfilling way to inspire others travelling a similar grief path. By openly discussing our personal growth or teaching lessons learned through grief, we create a ripple effect of healing that pays forward in a most satisfying way.

EMBRACING THE ONGOING JOURNEY

In the wake of grief, personal growth and transformation are not finite processes. On this ongoing journey, we evolve and adapt to the complexities of life. Grief itself is a lifelong process. It ebbs and flows with the passage of time. From it can emergence transformative life events experiences.

This journey of ebbs and flows is best navigated with resilience. We'll encounter moments of profound growth and insight, as well as periods of stagnation or regression. By accepting these fluctuations as natural parts of the healing process, we can cultivate patience. With grace, we can allow ourselves the space to fully experience our grief to integrate the lessons it provides.

Personal growth and transformation are not linear processes. Multidimensional experiences encompass various aspects of our lives—emotional, spiritual, psychological, and physical. With openness and curiosity, we will uncover new layers of meaning, purpose, and self-discovery, even years after our initial experiences of loss.

Grief is a profound, universal experience that can shatter our assumptions about life. It often shakes the very foundations of our existence. And yet, within this darkness lies the potential for profound transformation. Despite all its pain, grief is a catalyst for personal growth, self-discovery, and the cultivation of deeper meaning and purpose.

Ultimately, the transformative power of grief lies in its ability to awaken us to the preciousness of life. It can inspire us to live with greater meaning, purpose, and gratitude. For those who embrace this journey with an open heart and a curious spirit, the rewards are immeasurable. By embracing the lessons gained through loss, we can emerge not only intact, but truly transformed.

CHAPTER 13

SUPPORTING OTHERS

URING THE DARKEST MOMENTS OF grief, the support we receive from others can serve as our lifeline. Once we've experienced the depths of grief ourselves, we possess unique wisdom that often stirs empathy. That deep understanding of the complexities of loss is invaluable in supporting others on their own journeys of healing.

Drawing from personal experiences, we have the power to offer a level of compassion and insight that can help others feel seen, understood, and supported. By sharing our stories and lessons learned, we can be a beacon of hope. Our very presence among the grieving attests to the potential to heal.

Even if you choose not to become a mentor or grief counselor, you can use your experiences with grief to provide meaningful support to others behind you on the grief path. As a loved one, friend, or colleague, you can support those around you dealing with grief.

UNDERSTANDING THE GRIEVING PROCESS

Effectively supporting those who grieve requires a deep understanding of the grieving process itself. No two people experience grief exactly the same way. Even if another person loses a spouse to the same terminal illness that took yours, you cannot fully comprehend how they feel. No matter how similar your circumstances may seem, you will both experience grief uniquely. Hence, models and theories can provide only a framework for understanding the common stages and experiences of grief. But each person's journey is different. Personal circumstances, different coping mechanisms, and the unique nature of their loss all conspire to make their journey through grief like no other.

A key aspect of understanding the grieving process is acknowledging the non-linear and often cyclical nature of grief. It is not a straightforward progression from one stage to the next, but rather a constantly evolving, fluid experience with emotions ebbing and flowing like the tides. There may be moments of profound sadness, anger, or even guilt interspersed with periods of relative calm or acceptance.

To normalize them, it is important to validate the range of emotions and experiences that individuals may encounter during their grief journeys. From the intense pain and longing associated with loss, to the more complex emotions like relief, guilt, or even joy, each feeling deserves to be acknowledged so it can be processed.

By developing a deep understanding of the grieving process, we can better support those who grieve by providing a compassionate, non-judgmental space for them to express their emotions freely without fear of being misunderstood or invalidated.

EMPATHY AND ACTIVE LISTENING

At the heart of supporting others through grief lies the practice of empathy and active listening. Empathy is the ability to deeply understand, perhaps even share the feelings of another. We metaphorically step into their shoes to experience the world from their perspective. In the context of grief support, empathy involves creating a safe and non-judgmental space where individuals can freely express their emotions, thoughts, and experiences without fear of being dismissed or misunderstood.

Cultivating empathy requires us to develop emotional intelligence, self-awareness, and a willingness to truly listen without preconceived notions or personal biases. By suspending our own assumptions and judgments, we can seek to understand the unique perspectives of the person we are supporting.

Empaths must master active listening, which requires us to fully engage with the speaker. Non-verbally, we maintain eye contact or nod supportively. Verbally, we respond affirmatively to demonstrate our attentiveness and understanding. Even further, we can ask thoughtful questions that encourage deeper exploration and reflection, without imposing our own perspectives or solutions.

By practicing empathy through active listening, we can help the grieving feel validated and understood. As we provide a safe haven so the grieving can express emotions without fear of judgment, we invite them to explore and process their grief.

SHARING YOUR STORY

Sharing our own story is one of the most powerful tools to support the grieving. Our open vulnerably can create a deep sense of connection and understanding that transcends mere words.

Sharing personal experiences requires us to strike a delicate balance between providing insight and validation, while also allowing space for the other person's unique journey to unfold. The goal is not to impose our own experiences or perspectives, but rather to offer a window into the depths of grief and the potential for growth and healing that lies beyond.

Storytelling can be a potent tool in this regard, as it allows individuals to weave their experiences into a narrative that resonates on a deeper emotional level. Telling stories of the challenges we faced may spark hope or inspiration for those who are just beginning their own journeys. When we share the lessons they learned, we give the grieving a glimpse into transformative moments that can light the way toward healing.

Sharing stories requires discernment. We should be mindful of the timing, context, and emotional state of the persons we support. Sometimes our sharing deeply personal experiences could be overwhelming or triggering to the listener. In those instances, we can instead serve as a compassionate presence.

OFFERING PRACTICAL SUPPORT

While emotional support is undoubtedly a critical aspect of helping others through grief, it is equally important to address the practical challenges that often accompany loss. From navigating logistical complexities and decision-making, to coordinating support networks and accessing resources, there are numerous ways we can offer tangible assistance during this difficult time.

Helping them address logistical needs can help significantly, especially when they're at their most vulnerable. We might assist with funeral arrangements, help them manage legal or financial matters, or coordinate the distribution of personal belongings. For many who are grieving, these practical considerations can feel overwhelming. Our assistance takes some of the burden from them.

At a deeper level, we can help them with some decision-making. Grief can often cloud judgment and make it difficult to think clearly or weigh options objectively. As a non-judgmental sounding board who provides objective perspectives, we help the grieving make informed decisions that align with their values and the wishes of their loved ones.

Coordinating support networks and connecting individuals with available resources is a crucial form of practical assistance. Sometimes we may reach out to family members, friends, or community organizations to coordinate efforts and ensure that the individual's needs are being met comprehensively. We could also research and share information about support groups, counseling services, or other specialized resources that can aid in the healing process.

Our practical support alleviates some of the overwhelming challenges that often accompany grief. Such help allows the grieving to focus on their emotional and spiritual healing.

EMOTIONAL SUPPORT AND COPING STRATEGIES

While practical support is undoubtedly important, the emotional and psychological aspects of grief often require specialized care. After we have personally navigated the depths of loss, we're in a position to offer invaluable guidance. Even if the details of our grief differ vastly, the coping strategies we developed along the way could serve the people we're helping.

One of the most significant forms of emotional support is simply providing a safe, non-judgmental space for the grieving to express their emotions freely. This may involve actively listening, validating their feelings, and reminding them that their experiences are valid and normal.

In addition to creating a supportive environment, we can share coping strategies and self-care practices that helped us through our own grief journeys. Whenever we recognize that professional support may be needed, we can gently encourage them to seek counseling or join a support group. While our personal support can be invaluable, there may be times when they need the guidance of a trained professional to overcome particularly challenging experiences.

Throughout the emotional support process, we must approach each individual with empathy, patience, and a deep respect for the uniqueness of their journey. As a guiding light, we can remind them that healing is a process that includes even the darkest moments. Our presence attests to the value of tried and tested strategies for healing.

NAVIGATING DIFFICULT CONVERSATIONS

Supporting others through grief includes having difficult conversations that requires us to address sensitive topics with care and compassion. From discussing the circumstances surrounding a loved one's passing, to exploring complex emotions like guilt, anger, or regret, these conversations require a delicate touch drawn from a deep well of emotional intelligence.

Sometimes the most challenging aspect of these conversations is creating the space for them to occur. When feeling isolated by their grief, they may withdraw. With patience and gentle persistence, we can encourage them to open up and share their experiences.

When difficult conversations do arise, approach them with empathy, sensitivity, and a non-judgmental attitude. We can do that by actively listening, validating emotions, and assuring them they can express themselves freely, without fear of being dismissed or criticized.

We must be prepared to respond to common concerns and fears that may arise during these conversations. For example, individuals may express feelings of guilt or regret over things left unresolved with their loved one. In these instances, simply reminding them that grief is a complex, often irrational experience can validate their feelings and help them set a new course toward healing.

Throughout these conversations, maintain healthy boundaries and manage expectations. While providing emotional support is important, we must recognize the limits of our own expertise. When we see professional support is needed, we should have at our disposal additional resources or counseling opportunities for the grieving to pursue.

SUPPORTING SPECIFIC POPULATIONS

While grief is a universal experience, different populations may have unique needs and considerations when it comes to receiving support. From cultural and religious backgrounds to age and life stages, these factors can shape the grieving process and influence the most effective ways to provide support.

For example, we can best support individuals from diverse cultural or religious backgrounds by approaching their grief with sensitivity and respecting their traditions. This may involve educating ourselves on cultural practices surrounding death and mourning or seeking guidance from community leaders or elders to ensure we provide appropriate support.

Similarly, to support grieving youth requires an approach tailored to their cognitive and emotional development, as well as their specific needs and vulnerabilities. We may need to learn age-appropriate language or activities to help them process their emotions or secure the support of school counselors or child psychologists.

When supporting elderly individuals, be mindful of potential physical or cognitive limitations, as well as the unique challenges that can accompany grief in later life stages. This may involve coordinating additional support services, addressing concerns about loneliness or isolation, or navigating complex family dynamics.

Regardless of the specific population being supported, we can approach each individual with a deep sense of empathy, respect, and a willingness to learn and adapt. By seeking out resources, educating ourselves, and collaborating with professionals or community members who have specialized knowledge and expertise, we can ensure that our support is tailored, inclusive, and responsive to the unique needs of those we serve.

SELF-CARE AND BOUNDARY-SETTING

While supporting others through grief can be incredibly rewarding, this work also takes an emotional toll on us. Bearing witness to the depths of human suffering and holding space for intense emotions can drain and overwhelm anyone, even if we've traversed this region on our own grief journeys.

To ensure longevity and avoid burnout, prioritize self-care and establish healthy boundaries. This may involve setting aside dedicated time for rest and rejuvenation, engaging in activities that promote physical and emotional well-being, or seeking support from loved ones or professionals when needed.

A key aspect of self-care is learning to recognize and honor personal limits. While our desire to support others can be strong, we must know our own limits with emotional labor. It is sometimes necessary to say "no" to certain requests. We are also well-served to set clear boundaries around the time and energy we devote to supporting others.

It is also helpful to develop strategies for processing and releasing the emotional weight that can accumulate from holding space for others' grief. Practices such as journaling, meditating, or seeking professional counseling often work in this context.

By prioritizing self-care and boundary-setting, we are better able to show up fully present and emotionally available for those we support without sacrificing our own well-being in the process.

BUILDING A SUPPORT NETWORK

While personal support can be invaluable for the grieving, no one individual can provide all the support that may be needed. Building a broader support network, involving family, friends, community resources, and professionals, can help ensure that individuals receive comprehensive and holistic care during this challenging time.

Building a support network requires involving close family members and friends who can provide both practical and emotional assistance. To coordinate this effort, you may delegate tasks to ensure the griever's needs are being met in a consistent and cohesive manner.

Connecting individuals with support groups and community resources can be incredibly beneficial. Support groups allow participants to connect with others facing similar experiences. Community resources, such as religious organizations, non-profits, or local support services, can offer additional support.

Collaborating with professionals, such as counselors, therapists, or social workers, creates a comprehensive support network. These individuals can provide specialized expertise in areas such as grief counseling, trauma support, or navigating complex family dynamics.

Building a strong support network requires open communication, coordination, and a willingness to work collaboratively towards the shared goal of supporting the individual's healing journey. Leveraging the strengths and resources of various individuals and organizations is a comprehensive approach to support helps those in need without unduly taxing any one helper.

THE HEALING POWER OF HELPING OTHERS

While the primary focus of support is often on the individual who is grieving, we can find healing power by helping others navigate their own journeys of loss.

If you've experienced grief yourself, supporting others can also create new meaning and purpose for you. By sharing your experiences, insights, and hard-won wisdom, you can honor the memory of your loved ones and create a lasting legacy of hope and resilience.

Helping others can also promote personal growth and continued healing. As you share your stories and offer support, you may gain new perspectives on your own grief journey, uncovering layers of understanding or finding closure on lingering aspects of your own experiences.

Moreover, the reciprocal nature of support can create a profound sense of connection and community. By walking alongside others in their grief, you may find solace in the shared understanding that you are not alone, and that your experiences and struggles are part of the universal human experience.

Ultimately, the healing power of helping others lies in the recognition that grief, while profoundly personal, is also a shared journey that connects us all. By reaching out and offering support, we can not only aid in the healing of others, but also continue our own processes of growth, transformation, and the cultivation of meaning and purpose in the wake of loss.

Fundamentally, supporting others through the depths of grief is a sacred act. It requires empathy, courage, and a deep well of compassion. For those who have walked the path of loss themselves, their personal experiences can serve as a powerful source of wisdom and insight. They can be a guiding light for those just beginning their own journeys of healing.

Ultimately, the true power of supporting others lies in the ripple effect it can create. By offering compassionate guidance to those in need, we honor the memory of our loved ones by also contributing to a broader culture of healing.

As we continue to navigate the complex terrain of grief, may we all find the courage to reach out and offer support to those around us. In doing so, may we discover the profound healing power that comes from helping others and the deep sense of meaning and purpose that can emerge from even the darkest of life's journeys.

CHAPTER 14

PERSONAL PROGRESS

A s I APPROACH THE CONCLUSION of this book, I feel compelled to share my innermost thoughts and emotions from a personal perspective. Instead of merely describing experiences, I have decided to record my reflections and have them transcribed into written words. These intimate musings offer an unfiltered and genuine account of my journey.

Throughout this process, I have made some profound realizations that were seemingly apparent yet remained unacknowledged until now. I had not truly opened the door to my thoughts, feelings, and spoken words, expressing what I was observing and experiencing. It is crucial for me to capture these revelations and share them with you, my readers.

The timing holds great significance. Three years have passed since Debra's passing. The time feels both fleeting and eternal. Lonely weekends persist. The cherished bedtime hugs and cuddles are still sorely missed. Discussing the time I had with my beloved wife and best friend, as well as the time I wished we had but will never experience, still evokes deep emotions within me. Her passing on February 6th, 2021 marks the third year without her presence, a reality that remains difficult to fathom. The calendar's special dates—anniversaries, birthdays, Christmas, Easter—once joyous occasions, now unleash a torrent of emotions that can be challenging to manage. I have endured numerous trials and triumphs throughout this period, sometimes managing better than anticipated, while at other times, grief and sorrow have overwhelmed me.

SOCIETY AND COUPLES

One observation that continues to resonate and gain validation is realizing that much of society revolves around couples. It is structured to accommodate and prioritize the needs and experiences of couples rather than individuals who are single. The prevailing belief is that our purpose in life is to find our soulmate, that one special person with whom we will spend the rest of our lives.

However, life often throws unexpected circumstances our way. Sometimes, our soulmate leaves this world, leaving us feeling lost and alone.

Dealing with this situation has been one of the most challenging aspects for me, evoking a sense of being the odd one out, like a fifth wheel. Activities and social gatherings are often geared towards couples, which can make it difficult for those who are grieving. I perceive a constant focus on couples, be it at family dinners or other events. It's challenging for both the grieving individual and the well-meaning individuals who want to be inclusive but are unsure how to approach the situation.

COMMUNICATION

People often don't know how to handle grief or what to say when they encounter someone who has experienced loss. They may feel uncertain about how to approach the situation. In such instances, I've always appreciated it when someone is willing to ask me directly, seeking guidance on how they can support me. Instead of making assumptions, a simple inquiry can go a long way in showing genuine care and empathy. For example, one could say, "Doug, I find myself unsure of the right words to say, but I sincerely ask for your help in understanding how I could offer support."

I also often reflect on the celebration of life we held for Debra, and it remains a cherished memory. It was a truly remarkable event, filled with the presence of incredible individuals who shared their fondest memories of Debra. The opportunity to share those heartfelt stories with family, close friends, and others in attendance brought immense upliftment during what could have been a time dominated by immense sadness.

COMMITMENT

However, what struck me as interesting was the aftermath of such gatherings. Some individuals would approach me and express a desire to go out for lunch together, suggesting that we should make plans to connect. Naturally, I would agree and tell them to give me a call to arrange it. Sadly, as you might have anticipated, those calls never came. It is a recurring pattern I have observed. This experience has led me to emphasize the importance of following through on commitments, especially when offering support to someone dealing with grief. If you make a promise to meet for a meal or a cup of coffee, I urge you to honor it without delay. Such gestures hold tremendous significance.

When someone extends an invitation, it ignites a spark of anticipation within me. The prospect of stepping outside of my home, enjoying a conversation over coffee, or selecting a restaurant for a shared lunch becomes a source of genuine excitement. When these plans fall through, it leaves me questioning myself, wondering if I have done something wrong or if there was something more I could have done to make them feel at ease. It can be disheartening to have these opportunities taken away simply because someone is unsure of what to say or how to act.

Yet, I am grateful for the remarkable individuals who go above and beyond. All I need to do is pick up the phone and call, and we're off to the coffee shop for a coffee, shared tears, laughter, and a sense of companionship that sustains me until our next meeting.

Doug Lawrence

BEREAVEMENT SUPPORT

Participating in a bereavement support group has been a significant blessing. It has been truly therapeutic. I am grateful for the opportunity to serve as a volunteer alongside an extraordinary woman who leads this program. She has been a gift from above, as this group has been instrumental in helping me navigate challenging moments. Not only has it provided me with a support network, but it has also introduced me to various healing journeys and modalities that have proven immensely beneficial. Witnessing the profound impact this remarkable woman has had on me and others attending the group sessions has been truly awe-inspiring.

During my journey of grief, I've had encounters with various individuals, both virtually and in person. While I haven't had the opportunity to engage in significant conversations or share a coffee with them, these chance meetings serve as a reminder of the unpredictable nature of life. It is essential to embrace these encounters rather than inadvertently shunning them, as they are a part of my healing journey and therapeutic.

THE RISE IN GRIEF

The rise in grief is the very reason behind the subtitle of my book, *The Silent Pandemic*. We are witnessing a surge in grief due to various factors such as deaths caused by influenza, cancer, and other illnesses. Cancer remains one of the leading causes of death. Each loss gives rise to a unique journey of grief that demands attention and support.

Unfortunately, our collective ability to address and handle grief falls short of what it should be, thus earning it the designation of a silent pandemic. It is imperative that we establish robust support structures and provide the necessary assistance to those in need. One way to fortify such support systems is by incorporating mentoring, as discussed earlier in the book within the context of mental health. Grief is an integral part of mental health and should also be addressed within the support structures we establish.

One aspect I would like to mention is that most encounters I have these days seem to involve discussions or glimpses into the

realm of grief. It often overshadows other topics and presents itself in various forms, whether it be grief caused by the loss of a loved one or the challenges individuals face in terms of mental health.

NEW TRADITIONS

It's important to establish new traditions. Think back to some of the things you did with your loved one that held special meaning. In my case with Debra, she had certain traditions that she upheld every year, like our Christmas Eve gathering with signature cocktails and appetizers. We would have a pre-Christmas Eve taste testing to identify which drinks would be the signature cocktails for that year. While we still play games, we no longer do the pre-tasting, and I no longer have Debra's famous appetizers that everyone eagerly anticipated.

I have tried to make some of these traditions my own. For instance, I tend to go to bed a little earlier than Debra would have. I sense that this tradition is about to undergo yet another iteration, as the extended family appears to be wanting to create their own traditions. It's an important point I want to emphasize: you need to put into practice new traditions that will help you start the next chapter in your life story. Doing so will make a difference. Those traditions need to embrace love, happiness, and healing.

Your grief can come from many different sources—the loss of a loved one, the loss of a friend, job loss, or even the loss of your sense of self. You may find yourself asking, "What's in store for me tomorrow? What's in store for me the next day? Will I get from where I am today to where I think I want to be tomorrow?" All of that constitutes a form of loss. With that loss comes grief that you need to be able to address.

I have extensively discussed grief manifesting in various ways in the book—sadness, anger, denial, guilt, to name a few. I'm still struggling with many of these emotions. There are times of sadness and anger that everything happened the way it did. There is disappointment that I couldn't do more, and a lingering question of what I could have done differently to change the outcome. I keep contemplating the idea of swapping places with Debra, a notion that speaks to my need to find a way to manage these emotions without being consumed by them.

Another aspect that has become increasingly prevalent is the loss of family members, pets—our fur babies, our fur children, our grandchildren, as we affectionately call them. I have experienced this firsthand, going through the loss of two family pets in a relatively short timeframe. It's no different whether they have four legs or two. The feeling of loss is still the same. We still go through a process of grieving because they are part of our family, and we treat them as such. I have experienced both sides of this coin. Every time we had a family gathering before their passing, they were typically in attendance. After their loss, I noticed a gap, a void; they were no longer there to share those moments with us.

That empty feeling, the one I've talked about before, is particularly poignant when I reflect on the Christmas season. This past year, for some reason, I found it very difficult. A large part of it was because there is this huge void, this overwhelming feeling of emptiness and sadness that persists even three years after Debra's passing.

CONSIDERATIONS ABOUT THE PANDEMIC

Now I find myself asking, what truly constitutes a pandemic? From my perspective, cancer is a pandemic. Mental health, if we don't address it, is a pandemic that will continue to worsen, potentially leading individuals to take their own lives as a result of not being able to access the help they need to cope. Even with grief, there is a limit to how much one can endure before things have to change.

One challenging aspect I've encountered is receiving messages, whether by phone or mail, addressed to Debra. In one particular instance, it was the second time an organization called asking to speak with her. I explained the first time that it was not possible as she had passed away. Yet, the message never seemed to have been relayed, and they called again. I lost my voice, devastated. I had reached a point where I was managing reasonably well, but this felt like opening Pandora's box, triggering flashbacks and memories. Some involved work Debra was involved with, transporting me back to the countless times she would be late coming home because she was dealing with those issues, or when she would have to take off for a conference or other work-related obligations. All of those memories came flooding back.

WHO HELPS THE HEALER?

I was recently asked a thought-provoking question: As a mentor navigating the grieving process, how do you help others? It's a valid inquiry because ideally, every time you try to help someone, it can act as a trigger for your own grief.

A significant part of addressing this is leveraging the opportunity to have open conversations about how things are going for you at that moment. At the end of such a discussion, you can acknowledge, "I heard everything you said, and I saw myself in some of those instances. Talking with you is helping me figure out how I might deal with some of those situations that you're experiencing. I think I am experiencing it as well."

HOW DO I PROCESS MY TRAUMA? WHAT ARE MY COPING MECHANISMS?

I find myself grappling with questions like, "What do I consider to be trauma? Have I truly shed the trauma I experienced from my previous career?" The trauma fueled by my lived experiences from my past career, and even my current one, which included investigating loss of life, bullying, spousal abuse, alcoholism, and the constant change in our circle of friends, has forced me to be mindful that some of what I was experiencing—the trauma I was dealing with—was now closer to home than I ever imagined.

My use of alcohol, for example, as a coping mechanism for work-related trauma and grief, was making things worse. A large part of that stemmed from the nature of my job, which required me to be mobile and relocate to different locations based on the need for my services. My wife, Debra, and our two children would have to start over each time we relocated, meaning a new circle of friends and a new environment, some positive and some negative. There were times when, as police officers in certain communities, we would have to escort our wives to the grocery store. If we didn't, they became targets for physical and mental abuse.

One aspect that has been particularly triggering for me is the discussion of abuse against women and spousal abuse. I had a very close relationship with my mom, and hearing or even talking about these issues has been a huge trigger, as I'm always thinking of her, especially around the beginning of July when I make the journey back to our old home site and the cemetery where she and my dad are laid to rest. Debra would accompany me on this trip, during which I would clean up their grave sites. The journey itself is a significant trigger. The same can be said about how those particular triggers, especially spousal abuse, could have affected my relationship with Debra as well. Fortunately, we worked through any issues by communicating openly, ensuring we never had to deal with spousal abuse or violence. However, the triggers still linger.

SHARE YOUR FEELINGS

Whether it's grief or mental health, you must share your feelings. We've discussed this before: you need to share your thoughts and feelings and not keep them bottled up inside. By openly talking about them, you can engage in a healing therapy that you need. Don't feel pressured or pushed. Moving forward happens at the pace you decide, not according to someone else's timeline. You need to decide when you want to move forward.

As I approach the conclusion of this book, I want to emphasize that the journey we are embarking on together is lengthy, and it may not completely diminish the impact of grief. Many of the strategies I discussed can help alleviate grief to some extent. Whether you have acquired a copy of the book and have read a significant portion, including this final section, or if you have jumped to the end, I find engaging in conversations therapeutic, particularly with individuals who have experienced grief or are confronting mental health challenges. Sharing your story without fear or hesitation can be one of the most therapeutic actions you can take, truly making a world of difference and shaping the trajectory of your personal journey through grief.

In addition to practicing self-care, it is crucial to express your thoughts and emotions to someone who genuinely cares about your well-being. My sincere desire is for you to find solace and healing. Thank you for being a part of this journey. Thank you for acquiring a copy of *Grief: The Silent Pandemic.* If at any point you feel the need to reach out and have a conversation, please do not hesitate to do so. Contact information is provided within the book, including my website at www.talentc.ca, where you can find more information and reach out via email at doug.lawrence@talentc.ca. You can also find me on LinkedIn. Search my name, and my profile should appear. Once again, I express my gratitude, and I wish you all the best. Take care!

CONCLUSION

T HE INTRICATE RELATIONSHIP BETWEEN GRIEF and mental health confirms the urgency of addressing this silent pandemic. Losing a loved one is a universal human experience. Yet the depths of its impact on our mental well-being have long been underestimated and unaddressed. This book has sought to shed light on this critical issue, providing a comprehensive examination of the many ways grief can shape our emotional, psychological, and social lives.

Grief is a complex and multifaceted experience, one that defies simple categorization or linear progression. From the initial shock and denial to the eventual acceptance and integration, the journey of grief is a deeply personal one, shaped by individual circumstances, cultural contexts, and support systems. We have explored the various stages of grief, not as a rigid framework, but as a guide to understanding the common experiences and challenges that many individuals face in the wake of loss.

Moreover, grief can intersect with and compound other mental health challenges, such as depression, anxiety, and trauma. The loss of a loved one can be a triggering event, resurfacing past wounds and creating new ones. When left unaddressed, these challenges can lead to a downward spiral, impacting every aspect of an individual's life and well-being.

However, many pathways to healing and resilience exist for those who are grieving. The power of seeking support, whether through professional counseling, peer groups, or the guidance of a compassionate mentor, cannot be overstated. These connections provide a lifeline, reminding us that we are not alone in our struggles and that there is hope for healing and growth.

Mentoring, in particular, is central to working through grief. When an individual who has walked the path of grief before offers their wisdom, empathy, and guidance to someone who is currently struggling, it can be a transformative experience. Mentors can provide a safe space for processing difficult emotions, offer practical coping strategies, and serve as a model for resilience and growth.

Grief can impact different populations and contexts, from the unique challenges faced by youth to the need for greater support in the workplace. We must employ culturally sensitive and trauma-informed approaches to grief support, recognizing the diverse ways in which individuals and communities experience and express their loss.

Clearly, addressing the silent pandemic of grief and mental health demands a collective effort. We must shift our cultural attitudes and priorities with a willingness to confront the stigma and silence that have long surrounded these issues. It requires an investment in mental health resources and support systems, ensuring that everyone who is struggling has access to the care and compassion they need.

At the same time, it asks each of us, as individuals and as members of our communities, to play a role in creating a culture of openness, empathy, and understanding around grief and mental health. Whether by sharing our own stories, offering support to others, or advocating for change, we all have a part to play in breaking the silence and fostering healing.

The journey ahead may not be an easy one, but it is a necessary one. For too long, the pain of grief and the struggles of mental health have been borne in isolation, shrouded in shame and secrecy. There is power in bringing these experiences into the light, in connecting with others who understand, and in working together towards a world where no one has to suffer alone.

Beyond understanding the silent pandemic of grief and mental health, we must find the courage and compassion to face it head-on. Let us honor the loved ones we have lost, and the love that endures beyond their passing. We can recognize the strength and resilience that lies within each of us, even in the face of unimaginable pain.

As we step forward into the world, let us do so with a renewed commitment to prioritizing mental health, supporting those who are grieving, and creating a society where healing and hope can thrive.

The road ahead may be long, but every step we take brings us closer to a future where the silent pandemic is silent no more. Let us walk this path together, guided by the light of compassion, empathy, and the unbreakable bonds of human connection.

REFERENCES

Kübler-Ross, E. (1969). *On Death and Dying.* New York: Macmillan.

World Health Organization. (2022). Mental health and substance use. Retrieved from https://www.who.int/teams/mental-health-and-substance-use/overview

National Mentoring Resource Center. (2016). Mentoring for Youth with Mental Health Challenges. Retrieved from https://nationalmentoringresourcecenter.org/resource/mentoring-for-youth-with-mental-health-challenges/

ABOUT THE AUTHOR

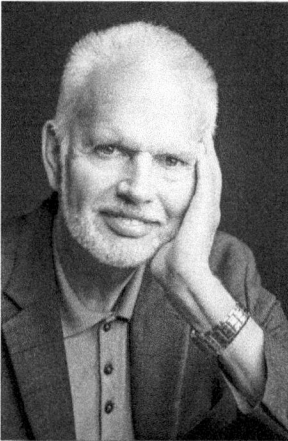

Doug Lawrence is the founder of TalentC® and is focused on all things mentoring as a solution provider. He is an International Certified Mentor who holds two Mentor Certifications: Certificate of Practice – Mentor and Certificate of Practice – Journey Mentor from the International Mentoring Community. Doug is the only one to hold the Certificate of Practice – Journey Mentor in the world today.

With over 30 years of mentoring and leadership experience, he is recognized as a thought leader in the mentoring space. He is also an international bestselling author. Doug's first book is *The Gift of Mentoring*. His second, *You Are Not Alone,* became an Amazon #1 Best Seller in North America and the UK. It earned a Bronze medal from the Global Book Awards.

Doug's Practice of Mentoring continues to grow and includes his work in dealing with grief and mental health. It has resulted in his accumulation of 3,400 hours of (in person and virtual) mentoring,

235 hours of public speaking, and 672 hours teaching others how to effectively mentor. In the past year, Doug has guest starred on approximately 150 podcasts sharing his wisdom about mentoring, mental health, and grief.